For Hoppy. Forever.

Thoughts of a Wild Pig
© 2025 Bind Publishing
All rights reserved.

First published in 2025 by Oli Hop
Manchester

ISBN: 9781036929190

Cover design by Oli Hop
Interior design and layout by Oli Hop
Printed in United Kingdom

This is a work of creative non-fiction. While based on personal experience, some names and identifying details have been changed to respect privacy.

For more information, visit: bind.co.uk

Thoughts of a Wild Pig
By Oli Hop

Part 1 - Wake the Fuck Up

Part 2 - Build the Fire

Part 3 - Burn the Old Script

Part 4 - Master the Mind

Part 5 - Full Fucking Ownership

Part 6 - Legacy Mode

Foreword.

This isn't a self-help book.
Not in the way you're used to.
There's no sugar. No softly-lit mantras. No step-by-step blueprint to manifest your dream life through vibes and smoothies.
This book is a punch in the ribs with a hand outstretched.

It's for the ones tired of pretending - who've outgrown the echo chamber of polished advice and ready for something raw and real. It's for the person who knows there's more in the tank but keeps stalling on the same old lies -
"I'm just not ready."
"I need to feel inspired."

Fuck that.

You won't find cute affirmations here. You'll find a mirror. A challenge. A knife to cut the bullshit, and a torch to burn the old script.
This isn't about hype - it's about grit.
Owning your story, not sanitising it. Taking responsibility, not outsourcing it. Building something real, messy, and powerful - not just posting about it.

There are no secrets here. No facts you can't find elsewhere.
Some of it you'll hate. Some of it might sting enough to make you stop and rethink a few things.
Read it slow. Scribble in the margins. Fold the corners. Skip around.
And remember - I'm not a respected author.
I'm just a guy with some thoughts to share…

Part 1

WAKE THE FUCK UP

Thought 1
The Myth of Motivation.

Motivation is bullshit. There, I said it.
Like a fart in the wind it arrives unannounced, makes a dramatic entrance, hangs around just long enough to be noticed, and then disappears before you can do anything useful with it.
Poof.
Gone.

People worship motivation like it's some mythical, infinite fuel source. As if the right YouTube video or podcast episode will flip a switch in your brain and suddenly you're running marathons at 5am and building your seven-figure business by lunchtime.
The truth?
Getting motivated is the easiest con your brain plays on you.
It happens all the fucking time - especially around January 1st when there's a flash sale on self-improvement.

You know the scene…
You're half-cut, slouched on the couch, thumbing through Instagram.
Up pops a transformation reel.
Some dude went from depressed couch potato to shredded entrepreneur in six months.
Another one claws their way out of a financial hole and now lives in Bali writing haikus and sipping overpriced mushroom coffee.
And for a moment, something sparks inside you…

"Shit…
That could be me.
That guy's a human…
And I'm a human…"

The metaphorical penny drops.
Bonk.
Your internal monologue kicks into overdrive…

"Enough is enough!
That's it!
I'm done with this bullshit life.
I'm throwing the ice cream in the bin, deleting the Domino's app,
buying the best pair of running shoes money can buy, and writing my
bulletproof business plan with the smooth ink of a Montblanc pen."

You feel like a god.
You've signed a blood oath with yourself to finally become Version 2.0.
And for a little while…
It works.
You wake up earlier.
You eat like an influencer on a sponsored meal plan. You're laser
focused.
You're in 'the zone'.
But here's the kicker…
It.
Doesn't.
Last.
Motivation is a one-night stand with potential.
Whispers promises in the dark, then ghosts you with your pants round
your ankles and dreams half-dressed.

Friction Is the Killer.

Maybe it's a shitty night's sleep.
Or your partner hits you with a sideways comment that slices deeper
than it should.
Or maybe it's just raining and cold, and your Nikes are still soaked
from yesterday's efforts.
Whatever it is, that godlike momentum you were riding?
It fades quicker than a cokehead's clarity at 3am.

Suddenly everything feels hard.
Going to the gym feels like dragging a corpse.
Saying no to pizza feels like denying yourself oxygen.
Sitting down to map out that 'bulletproof' business plan feels like pure medieval torture.
Because the brain is a conniving little bastard.
The moment it senses discomfort, it starts clawing for the escape hatch. Anything to slip back into the warm, greasy hug of comfort.
Friction is the silent killer.
It doesn't stab you outright - it bores holes in your willpower until everything feels impossible.

The Biology of Self-Sabotage.

We're all dopamine junkies.
You, me, the postman - we're all riding the evolutionary rollercoaster of instant gratification.
Think of Eminem and Dr. Dre's track 'Guilty Conscience'.
The duo personify the devil and angel on a man's shoulders, each arguing over moral choices.
Dre is the voice of reason.
And Em?
He's temptation and instant gratification - urging the character toward destructive actions.
Crude?
Yes.
Accurate?
Fuck yes.
Because every single decision you make - whether it's kale or cake, reps or rest, ambition or apathy - that same showdown is playing out in your
head.
The devil is your impulsive side, hellbent on chasing the next dopamine
hit.
And the angel?
That faint, pitiful whisper asking you to think long-term.

To maybe not fuck up your future for five minutes of pleasure.
The problem is that every time you ignore the angel, its voice gets fainter, until it's just background noise you've learned to tune out.
So you break.
You reach for the hobnobs.
You skip the run.
You binge a series you've already seen.
You hand the wheel back to the old you, and sit there wondering why your life remains exactly the fucking same.

Your Expectation of Ease.

Motivation is cheap.
Discipline is expensive.
And because motivation feels good, like a hit of sugar to the soul, we start believing it should feel that way all the time.
Real transformation is different.
It's gritty.
It's repetitive.
It's boring as hell.
It's dragging yourself out of bed at 5:30 in the morning when you'd rather punch the snooze button.
It's dragging yourself to pound the pavement when your body's stiff and your mind's louder than your alarm.
It's working towards your goals when no one's watching, and no one cares.
That's the cost.
And most people are too broke in willpower to pay the price.
They want change to be cute and easy.
They want abs without sweat, cash without effort, success without mess.
But this isn't Amazon Prime.
You don't click 'get motivated' and have your dreams delivered by Tuesday.
You grind.
You bleed.
You show up anyway.

That's the difference between those who change their lives, and those who just change the wallpaper on their vision board.

From Motivation to Habit.

Here's the fix - you don't need better motivation, you need a better system.
Your job isn't to wait until you feel inspired.
Your job is to build a life where motivation becomes irrelevant.
You've got to make habits do the heavy lifting - because if your progress depends on your mood, you're already fucked.
Feelings lie.
Systems don't.
Habit is brushing your teeth without thinking.
Habit is putting your shoes on before your brain has a chance to complain.
Habit is doing the next right thing, even when it feels pointless.
You don't rise to the level of your goals, you fall to the strength of your patterns.
So build better patterns.
Then let those patterns build you.

Build Your Basement.

The problem with motivation is that it's a high.
And highs wear off.
If your life is built on hype videos and motivational quotes, it's going to collapse the second reality smacks you in the mouth.
But if your foundation is discipline, if you've built a basement of boring, consistent, automatic reps?
Then when the storm hits (and it will), you're ready.
You don't flinch.
You don't pause.
You don't perform a 'vibe check'.
You just do the thing.

Burn Your Motivation Journal.

Here's your truth bomb - motivation is for tourists.
Systems are for lifers.
And discipline is the bridge between who you are and who you want to be.
You're not lazy.
You're not broken.
You're not missing some secret gene.
You're just stuck on the rollercoaster of emotional highs and inevitable crash landings, because you've been brainwashed into thinking the only time to act is when you feel inspired.

Fuck that.

Feelings are charming liars.
You've got to build your day around actions, not emotions.
Let your identity come from follow-through, not feeling.
And for fuck sake, stop waiting to feel like it.
This is your green light to stop being a tourist in your own life.
Kill the quotes.
Bin the hype.
Ditch the dopamine circus.
Get boring.
Get brutal.
Get building.
Because nothing beats the person who shows up, shuts up, and does the work...
Even when the motivation's six feet under.

Put It On the Table.

Does this 'thought' hit home?
☐ Yes   ☐ Not really

If yes, can you call yourself out and apply it?
☐ Yes   ☐ Still hiding

If yes, what's one move you'll make to prove it's not just words?

....

....

Thought 2
You're the Problem - You're Also the Solution.

If you're not where you want to be in life, there's one truth you've got to swallow whole...
You are the common denominator.
The jobs that didn't work out.
The failed relationships.
The broken promises.
The plateaus, the stalls, the spirals - you were there for all of them.

Now, before you start moping and assume this is some cruel kick while you're down, pause.
This isn't an insult - it's an invitation.
Because the moment you admit you're the problem, you unlock the only truth that matters - you're also the fucking solution.

You're the Plug and the Power.

No mentor, no lover, no miracle plan is going to swoop in and fix your life for you.
If you're waiting for that, you're just handing away your power.
The second you stop blaming others, that's when shit starts to shift.
You take the wheel.
You stop being a passenger in your own life.
You start driving.

Blame Is a Drug.

Blame is addictive.
It gives you something to point at when things fall apart.
The dirty secret is that blame feels good because it removes your responsibility.
And that might keep your ego safe, but it keeps your life small.

People who point fingers don't build empires.
They build echo chambers.
Safe.
Stagnant.
Sterile.
And echo chambers don't grow - they decay.
They rot while you sit there, surrounded by excuses that sound smart, but keep you exactly where you are.
So if you're ready to grow, drop the blame.
Withdraw from the drug.
And start owning your shit like your future depends on it.

Extreme Ownership Is Where Power Starts.

If you're not taking ownership, you're not in control.
And if you're not in control, then your circumstances own you.
Own your decisions.
Own your inaction.
Own your attitude.
Own the fact that you let bullshit slide, played small, dodged hard truths, and settled when you should've stepped the fuck up.
This isn't self-hate - it's being honest enough to stop lying.

Radical honesty is the prerequisite for real change, and most people are allergic to it.
It's not about blame - it's about extreme ownership.
That means no more, *"I'll see how I feel."*
No more, *"I'm just not in the right headspace."*
No more pretending circumstances are stronger than your choices.

Because the truth is you built this life, piece by piece, choice by choice, conscious or not.
Which means you can tear it down.
Rebuild it.
Shape it like fucking clay.

You don't need more clarity - you need more courage.
You don't need a therapist to tell you what you already know - you need to act like your future depends on it.
Just guts.
Just grit.
Just the willingness to look in the mirror and say - "*This is mine. And I'm taking it back.*"

You're Not Stuck, You're Just Unwilling.

You say you want change, but you're still numbing out with distractions.
Still chasing likes instead of progress.
Still choosing comfort over your calling.
You're not stuck.
You're just repeating the same choices and hoping for different results.
The turning point is when you finally get tired of your own bullshit.

Real Change Is Built on Brutal Honesty.

Want to level up?
Start here...
"*Where am I getting in my own way?*"
Ask it without ego.
Answer it without excuses.
Then fix it without delay.
Your mindset, your discipline, your habits, your energy, your circle - they're all reflections of what you tolerate.
If they're not serving you, stop whining, and tweak the system.

You Need a New Standard.

Most people don't need a full reset.
They just need to raise the bar on what they accept from themselves.
Stop letting, "*It's not that bad*" be your baseline.
"*At least I'm better than X*" be your ceiling.

Set a new standard.
Then hold the fuck to it.
And when you slip, because you will, own it and get back up stronger.

The Bad News Is You. The Good News Is Also You.

This thought isn't about shame.
It's about power.
You made your own mess.
Cool.
You're also the only one qualified to clean it up.
You can change your mindset.
You can choose different inputs.
You can rebuild, repurpose, reinvent - starting right fucking now.
There's nothing more liberating than looking in the mirror and saying,
"*I'm the problem. I'm the solution. And I'm not waiting on anyone to fix me.*"
That's not defeat.
That's day one.

Put It On the Table.

Does this 'thought' hit home?
☐ Yes   ☐ Not really

If yes, can you call yourself out and apply it?
☐ Yes   ☐ Still hiding

If yes, what's one move you'll make to prove it's not just words?

....

....

Thought 3
Pigeonholes Are for Pigeons.

People love boxes.
      It helps them sleep at night.
But here's the problem - I don't fit in a fucking box.
I'm 6'6", 240 pounds.
Built like a grizzly that snacks on small children.
Covered in tattoos, bearded, and sweary.
Resting face of a thunderstorm.

I walk down the street, and people cross it.
Not a polite sidestep - I mean a full-blown Frogger across traffic like I'm holding a chainsaw.
It's surreal.
Like I'm radioactive - get too close and they'll spontaneously combust.
Most days, I shrug it off.
It's a survival instinct.
I get it, we all have it.
And let's face it, the world is full of cunts.

But every now and then it gets to me.
Like when I see a mum pushing a pram.
Or an old couple enjoying their slow, sacred shuffle.
That's when I'm the one that crosses the road.
Not because I'm a threat, but because I don't want them to feel afraid.
I carry the burden of their assumption so they don't have to.
They get to keep their comfort.
I get to swallow the stereotype.

And here's the punchline...
I.
Am.
Not.
A.
Terrorist.

Behind the Beard.

You see a big, tattooed, scowling bloke stomping down the pavement.
What you don't see is this...
That face that looks like I'm plotting your doom?
It's probably just me wrestling with a critical thought experiment -
...Would you rather fight 1000 duck-sized horses or one horse-sized duck?...
That's where I'm at mentally.
Not rage.
Not violence.
Just existential poultry math.

There's more you don't know...
I cry during the stampede in 'The Lion King'.
Every.
Damn.
Time.
I donate to charities when I can, even when my bank account wheezes on life support.
I once lived next door to a crack addict named Justin - our agreement was five cigarettes for one go on his washing machine.
I respected the trade - he respected the cycle.
Mutual respect.
Clean pants.
No drama.

And then there's my daughter.
My world.
The anchor in the storm.

The thing I look forward to most is reading with her.
Our go-to book?
'The Tiger Who Came to Tea'.
Certified banger.
Five stars.
Would recommend.
And yes, I'm convinced the cat you see on the penultimate page is the tiger in disguise.
Don't @ me - I'll die on that hill.

It's in My Blood.

My old man - Nick Hopkinson.
Known as Hoppy or Hoppyman.
The original gentle giant.
He was the size and shape of a Smeg fridge.
Hair like a haystack with unresolved trauma.
Dressed like Stig of the Dump crossed with Dame Edna.
But kindness was carved into his DNA.
Unbreakable, unshakable kindness.
And he knew exactly what people saw when they looked at him -
"Tramp."
"Weirdo."
"Threat."
So he leaned into it and used it as a filter.
If your first instinct was to judge him by how he looked?
Cool.
You just saved him the trouble of getting to know you.
You failed the test.
You saw the cover and didn't bother opening the book.

We all love to say, *"Don't judge a book by its cover."*
But let's be real - covers sell.
Designers obsess over them.
Test them.
Pick the right colour, font, finish - because deep down we all judge.
Same with products.

You buy the perfume in the tin can because the bottle looks cool.
That's it.
That's the logic.
Packaging over substance.
Form over function.
Surface over soul.
And you wonder why the world's so broken?

The Mental Health Mask.

Now we hit the raw nerve.
You know why there's a stigma around mental health?
Because we've been trained and conditioned to fear it.
You see it in films - the wild-eyed villain with a tragic backstory and a knife.
In the news, "*Man with mental health history...*" as if that explains everything.
Lazy storytelling.
Toxic assumptions.
Repeated until it becomes gospel.

So let's debunk some classic bullshittery -
"*People with mental illness are dangerous.*"
"*Depression is weakness.*"
"*Addiction is a choice.*"
"*Therapy is for the broken.*"
You know what that is?
Bullshit.
A steaming pile of bullshit.
Covered in bullshit.

Here's the truth...
Mental illness can look like the dad reading '*The Tiger Who Came to Tea*' for the 400th time.
It can look like the bloke who makes everyone laugh at the pub.
It can look like someone building a business, smashing targets, and going home to cry in the shower.

It can look like… me.

My Story.

In 2004, I shattered.
Not figuratively - I mean full, soul-level implosion.
Diagnosis?
A cocktail of depression, anxiety, PTSD and bipolar.
All the labels.
All at once.
I was fully fucked and moved back in with my parents.
I couldn't step outside without spiralling into a full-blown panic attack.
At one point, I genuinely believed I was dead.
A ghost.
Floating through life invisible, untouchable, forgotten.

Recovery?
It's still ongoing.
And that's okay.
Progress isn't linear.
Healing doesn't punch a clock.
But here's the thing -
Through my mental illness, I became better.
More self-aware.
More compassionate.
More patient with others - even the cunts.
Am I fragile?
Dangerous?
Less capable?
Fuck no.

Stop Judging the Package.

I won't list my creds.
If you need receipts to respect me, you're not my audience.
But I'll say this…

If you're the type to judge, stereotype, and write others off based on surface-level bullshit - may you trip and fall down a deep well.
Not out of cruelty.
Out of hope.
Hope that the silence down there gives you space to sit with yourself.
To ask real questions.
To maybe, just maybe, unlearn your bullshit.
Maybe you'll realise that you can't know a person by their beard or tattoos or posture or voice.
Maybe you'll finally understand - people are more than packaging.

We Are Not What You Assume.

We are contradictions wrapped in skin.
Wounded and healing.
Hard and soft.
Angry and loving.
Fierce protectors and fragile artists.
We're walking paradoxes.
Every single one of us.
So next time you catch yourself labelling someone - stop.
Because pigeonholes are for pigeons bro.

Put It On the Table.

Does this 'thought' hit home?
□ Yes   □ Not really

If yes, can you call yourself out and apply it?
□ Yes   □ Still hiding

If yes, what's one move you'll make to prove it's not just words?

....

....

Thought 4
The Universe Hates You.

The universe is against everything you do.
You come up with a plan?
The universe drafts 100 reasons why it won't work.
You crave change?
It sends 100 reminders that it's safer to stay the same.
You want something - anything?
Expect resistance, hurdles, dead ends, fog, fire, and flatlining motivation.
Because the universe doesn't want you to win.
It wants balance.
It's obsessed with equilibrium, like some cosmic bastard with a clipboard and a smug grin.
And here's the fucked up thing - I like that.
I like that it fights us.
Because it means everything we earn was fought for.
It means we grow.
We appreciate the mountain because we clawed our way up the fucker. And when you've dragged your tired, blistered body to the top, you don't just see the view.
You become the view.

And what got you there?
Not talent.
Not luck.
Not your morning affirmations.
Grit.
My favourite human trait.
Forget charm, forget potential - give me someone with grit and I'll show you someone dangerous.

In the best possible way.

Marathons and Broken Pencils.

Let's say you've got a dream.
Something big.
Something painful.
Something that makes you ache in your chest just thinking about it.
Like running a marathon.
26.2 miles of self-inflicted madness.
You've trained.
You're ready.
You've got the playlist, the gels, and *"Stay Hard"* sharpied onto your forearm.
But the universe?
It's waiting at mile 20.
And it's bringing cramp, self-doubt, and the sudden realisation that this was a fucking terrible idea.
You hit the wall.
You break.
You fail.
You feel like shit.

Now here's where it gets interesting - because this is where masks fall off.
Where the hype dies.
Where motivation runs out.
And all that's left is you.
Not the curated version, or the one who tweets discipline quotes.
The real one.

There are three kinds of people in this world -
1. Those who really try.
2. Those who don't.
And the most tragic kind of all,
3. Those who pretend to try...

The 80-percenters who call it 100.
The ones who build exits and label them detours.
The ones who had more to give but didn't.
Those people?
They're like broken pencils - pointless.
They get from A to F and then quit.
F for Fucked.

How to Beat the Universe (Kind Of).

Want a chance at beating the universe?
Here's the cheat code...
Try.
Not the Instagram kind of trying.
Not the "*I did a bit and hoped it stuck*" trying.
The real kind.
The sweaty, gritty, no witnesses kind.
The kind where you do the prep, anticipate where shit will fall apart,
and build like the storm is guaranteed.
The kind where you've built something so solid that when you hit the
wall, your legs keep moving.
The kind where, win or lose, you can go to bed at night, stare up at the
ceiling and say - "*I left nothing on the table.*"

The universe might still hit you.
It might bring curveballs, setbacks and last-minute sabotage.
But if you've put the work in?
You have a chance.
Maybe not a win.
But a worthy battle.

Let's throw in some algebra for my fellow numerophiles -

$$\text{Effort} - \text{Universe Resistance} = X$$

If X is positive?
You succeed.

If X is negative?
You fail.
Simples.

Failing Gracefully - The Underrated Art.

There's a twist...
Sometimes, you do everything right, and the universe still smacks you down.
You did the prep.
You did the work.
You followed every rule, X was positive, and still got blindsided.
Covid.
Car crash.
A rolled ankle.
Redundancy.
Sudden grief.
Life throws you a card you couldn't have seen coming.
And you fail.
But this time it's different.
This time you fail gracefully.
And that? That's fucking beautiful.

Failing gracefully means -
You showed up.
You fought hard.
You refused to lie to yourself.
You didn't sell out for the easy route.
And when you fall, you don't flounder.
You get up, dust off, and whisper - *"that was round one."*

Graceful failure is addictive.
It teaches you things a win never will.
It strengthens your character in the quietest, most unshakable ways.
The war isn't won or lost in one battle.
Lose the round, regroup, and reload.

The Universe's Secret Weapon.

Listen up, because this is where most people get fucked.
We've talked about how the universe resists you.
But you know what its most dangerous weapon is?
People.
Your colleagues, your friends, even your blood.
The world is full of haters, jealous wrecks, energy vampires in friendship form and small minds that fear ambition.
You could be making progress, working on yourself, chasing something real.
But if the people around you are dream-suckers?
You're fucked.
They can wreck you faster than failure ever could.
They're not cartoon villains.
They won't swing at you directly.
They'll bleed you in cunning ways - slowly, subtly, silently.

They don't even have to say much.
A sideways glance.
A sarcastic comment.
A lazy, *"Don't push yourself too hard"* wrapped in fake concern.
And just like that, your fire dims.
Not because you doubted yourself - but because someone else's fear got loud enough to drown out your courage.
That shit is lethal.
You need to protect your inner circle like your life depends on it - because it does.

The Right Ones Light Fires.

The right people don't let you quit.
They don't pity your pain - they respect it.
They see your suffering and say, *"This is proof you're on the right path."*
When you're dragging yourself through hell, they don't hand you a white towel - they walk beside you.

Their faith in you lights fires in places you didn't even know you had fuel left.
Surround yourself with people like that, people who remind you who the fuck you are when you forget, and suddenly the universe looks beatable.

Lone Wolves.

If the choice is between being a lone wolf and being surrounded by broken pencils...
Walk alone.
Any day.
Every day.
Because there's nothing lonelier than being surrounded by people who don't believe in you.
Or worse - people who only support the version of you that stays small.

So choose the silence of solitude over the noise of small minds.
And next time the universe shows up with resistance, cramp, and chaos...
Pop the kettle on. You've been expecting it.

Put It On the Table.

Does this 'thought' hit home?
☐ Yes   ☐ Not really

If yes, can you call yourself out and apply it?
☐ Yes   ☐ Still hiding

If yes, what's one move you'll make to prove it's not just words?

....

....

Thought 5
Self-Pity Is a Drug, and Most People Are Addicted.

Feeling sorry for yourself is easier than fixing it.
There's a sickness running through the world right now - and no one wants to call it what it is.
It's not burnout.
It's not trauma.
It's not 'the system'.
It's self-pity - and it's being snorted like a line of comfort in every corner of society.
Everyone wants to feel seen.
Everyone wants empathy.
But somewhere along the way, the line blurred between being understood and being enabled.

Victimhood Is the New Currency.

Play the victim, and the world opens its arms.
Sympathy rushes in.
You'll get claps for being brave.
Likes.
Nods.
"You're so strong."
All without having to take a single step forward.

And that's the trap.

Because self-pity feels good.
It wraps around you like a warm blanket and whispers, *"This isn't your fault. Stay here. You deserve to feel like this."*
But that blanket?
It's made of chains.

And while you're curled up in it, the world keeps spinning.
Opportunities keep moving.
Someone else is doing the shit you keep dreaming about.
While you're typing out another post about why the odds are stacked against you, someone else is stacking wins.

Yes, Life's Been Hard.

Everyone's got scars.
Everyone's been blindsided.
Everyone's taken hits they didn't deserve.
The cold truth is - no one's coming to save you.
The only question that matters is - what are you going to
do now that it's happened?

You can keep telling your story like a eulogy, or you can tell it like an origin story.
Because if you live in self-pity long enough, it starts renting space in your soul - and before you know it, it owns the fucking lease.
You build your entire identity around your pain.
You start thinking the world owes you comfort just because it once gave you hell.
Newsflash - it doesn't owe you shit.
But you owe yourself a comeback.

The False High.

Self-pity is narcotic comfort.
It feeds you drama, a hit of attention, and a nice rush of validation.
But like any drug, the comedown is brutal.

And the longer you stay high on it, the more it warps your reality.

You start measuring your worth in suffering.
You start competing in the Olympics of misery.
You start feeling attacked by people who've simply chosen to move on.
And when someone finally holds up a mirror instead of a tissue?
You call them toxic.
You say they don't understand.
You label truth as cruelty because comfort became your only compass.

The Fix Is Ugly.

Self-pity doesn't want you to move.
It wants you to sit and sulk.
To keep curating that sad little narrative where you're the passenger in your own life - and bad shit just *"happens to you."*

The antidote?
Movement.
Ownership.
Brutal self-respect.
Get up.
Get outside.
Do the thing you've been avoiding.
Call yourself out before someone else has to.
Stop bleeding on everyone who didn't cut you.
Stop weaponising your wounds like they excuse your inaction.
That's not being harsh.
That's called growing the fuck up.

Most People Don't Want Healing.

They say they want to heal - but what they really want is applause for being broken.

They want the likes.
The pity.
The comfort choir singing *"You're so strong"* just for showing up.
Because actual healing?
That shit takes work.
Hard, boring, repetitive work.

It's way easier to say, *"I've been through a lot,"* and let that be the full sentence.
A full stop.
A fucking identity badge.
But healing isn't a TED Talk or a mood board.
It's choosing growth over gossip.
It's showing up on the days you feel hollow.
It's dragging yourself back to the fight after the tears have dried and the sympathy's run out.
It's thankless.
It's gritty.
And it's the only way forward.

Pain Is Real, But So Is Choice.

This isn't about denying pain.
This is about reminding you that pain isn't the full story.
You don't get to skip the pain.
But you do get to choose what you do with it.
Let it rot you, or let it forge you.
Let it break your back, or build your backbone.

Some Karens reading this will flinch.
That's good.
The truth's meant to sting when you've been self-soothing too long.

Progress Doesn't Pander.

Want a pat on the back?

Go see a chiropractor.
Want transformation?
Get ready to bleed for it.
Progress doesn't hold your hand.
It slaps the excuses out of your mouth and makes you earn every step forward.
And most people can't stomach that.
They want six-pack results with marshmallow discipline.
They want success that never asks for sacrifice.

Progress is allergic to pity.
It doesn't give a fuck what you've been through - it only responds to what you're willing to do about it.

Pity Feels Safe. Power Feels Better.

Bad days?
Totally human.
Support?
Necessary.
Falling apart?
Sometimes inevitable.
But living there?..
Camping out in the wreckage and expecting a medal for surviving it?..
That's where growth goes to die.
Victims wait.
Fighters adapt.
Builders rise.

If you're reading this and feeling called out, that means your fight isn't dead.
It's just buried under bullshit.
So stand up.
Shake it off.
And start again - with your head up and your excuses in the bin.

Put It On the Table.

Does this 'thought' hit home?
☐ Yes   ☐ Not really

If yes, can you call yourself out and apply it?
☐ Yes   ☐ Still hiding

If yes, what's one move you'll make to prove it's not just words?

....

....

Thought 6
Log Off, You're Not a Fucking Algorithm.

I'm sick to death of this social media circus.
Sick of watching kids spiral into depression because their picture didn't get enough likes.
Sick of grown adults having identity crises over an unfollow.
Sick of seeing people tie their entire self-worth to comments, filters, and fucking engagement stats.

We've built a world where a selfie has more value than a conversation.
Where dopamine comes from double taps.
Where self-esteem is built on validation from strangers you wouldn't lend a fiver to in real life.
You think that's normal?
You think that's sustainable?

Let me say this as clearly as I can...
You weren't built to be liked.
You were built to live.
You are not a fucking algorithm.

Likes Don't Equal Love.

Likes don't mean shit.
They may look like little a thumbs-up or hearts, but they're not love.
They're not truth.
They're not real.

They're pixels and patterns engineered to keep you scrolling, comparing, and coming back for more.

You post a photo, it gets 3 likes, and suddenly you're questioning your whole existence.
You start thinking -
"Maybe I'm not attractive."
"Maybe no one cares."
"Maybe I'm just boring."
"Maybe I should delete it."

What the actual fuck are we doing?!

A generation raised on participation trophies is now being emotionally waterboarded by a machine that only rewards perceived perfection.
You're chasing high scores on a fake scoreboard.
And every time you lose, you blame yourself, not the game.

The Highlight Reel Is a Lie.

Social media isn't real life.
It's a highlight reel of everyone's best moments, edited to look like a lifestyle.
It's the airbrushed, filtered, curated version of someone else's fake-ass fairy tale.
You're comparing your behind-the-scenes chaos to someone else's staged performance.
That #couplegoals post?
They were screaming at each other an hour later.
That ripped gym bro?
Filtered to fuck, and juiced to the gills.
That happy entrepreneur?
Maxed-out credit cards and a panic disorder.

You're losing sleep over people lying for likes.
You're questioning your own life because someone else nailed their lighting setup.

Social media is a magic trick.
And you're letting the smoke and mirrors tell you how to feel about yourself?
Wake the fuck up.

Digital Validation Is a Drug.

Let's call it what it is - addiction.
Social media works like a casino - random rewards and intermittent dopamine hits.
Just enough attention to keep you hooked and hungry.
This isn't a weakness - it's a setup.
Your brain's been manipulated by something designed to exploit it.
But here's the scary part...
Unlike other addictions, this one is socially accepted.
Encouraged even.

Post more.
Share more.
Hustle harder.
Build your brand.
Grow your audience.
Fuck.
All.
Of.
That...
You're not a brand.
You're not a product.
You're not a fucking algorithm in sneakers.
You're a human.
Not a product.
Not a profile.
Not a follower count.
Not a piece of content.
Just a messy, raw, breathing human.
And you deserve to live like one.

Live Where Your Feet Are.

You want peace?
Freedom?
Confidence?
Get the fuck offline.
Log off.
Shut down.
Reboot your reality.

Live where your feet are, not in your followers list.
Not inside a comment section.
Not in an 'insight dashboard'.
Look people in the eyes, not their avatars.
Make memories, not content.
Go outside and do something beautiful without filming it.
Eat a meal without showing your plate to the world.
Have a moment, just for yourself.
No hashtags.
No filters.
No "tap to reveal more."
Just you.
Just… life.
And you'll be shocked at how rich it feels when it isn't flattened into an IG story.

The Ducks and the Tiger.

It took me 33 years to really learn this lesson.
Then it hit me like a fucking bus.
I was newly married, running on fumes, trying to keep a struggling tech business from flatlining.
I was living off perception - grinding hard, posting the hustle, desperate to look like I had my shit together.

One day, I took my 3-year-old daughter out for a walk so my wife could rest.

Nothing dramatic.
Just a quiet stroll.
We found a bench by a pond.
There were ducks.
We sat.
Fed them.
Read *'The Tiger Who Came to Tea'* - her favourite.
No camera.
No post.
No audience.
Just me, her, the ducks… and the tiger.
In that silence, that completely unshared, unfiltered, unbranded
moment - I thought, *"Fuck me. I'm lucky."*

Not because I had anything fancy.
But because I was fully present.
Alive in a moment that didn't need validation to be real.

That moment changed me.

Your Worth Isn't Measured in Metrics.

If you died tomorrow, Instagram wouldn't mourn you.
TikTok wouldn't flinch.
Facebook wouldn't blink.
But your people would.
The ones who've heard your real laugh.
The ones who've seen you cry without a filter.
The ones who don't need a like button to show love.
That's where your value lives - not in impressions, but in impact.
Not in how many watched, but in who remembers.

Step Outside the Screen.

One day, when you're old and wrinkled, you won't give a flying shit
how many people double-tapped your sunset pic.

You won't reminisce about your follower count.
You won't whisper analytics on your deathbed.
You'll care about the real stuff.
The laughs.
The bruises.
The love you felt without needing to post about it.
The adventures that didn't make it to your story, but etched themselves into your soul.
The real shit.
The shit that stayed.

So here's the move...
Step outside the screen.
And live like your battery's already dead.
Put your phone down.
Pick your life up.
And remember you're not here to be consumed.
You're here to be alive.

Put It On the Table.

Does this 'thought' hit home?
☐ Yes   ☐ Not really

If yes, can you call yourself out and apply it?
☐ Yes   ☐ Still hiding

If yes, what's one move you'll make to prove it's not just words?

....

....

Thought 7
You Can't Heal If You're Still Holding the Knife.

Everyone talks about growth like it's a gym membership.
Do the reps.
Drink the smoothie.
Read the book.
Rise and grind…
Cool story bro.
But no one talks about what comes before all that.
The rot under the floorboards.
The emotional mould that's been growing in silence.
The guilt.
The shame.
The echo of bad decisions that still lives in your chest like a parasite.
The voice that says - *"Who the fuck are you to change?"*

It's not always laziness holding you back.
Sometimes it's punishment.
And you're the one swinging the hammer.

The Hardest Person to Forgive Is Yourself.

Maybe you hurt someone.
Maybe you wasted years doing the wrong thing.
Maybe you burned bridges or let someone down or drowned your potential in a bottle, a lie, or a habit you swore you'd kick.

And now you're trying to build a new life on top of that foundation.

But you never cleared the rubble.
You're stacking goals, habits, and grindsets on top of shame that hasn't been dealt with.
The truth is you can't build something strong when your foundation is cracked by guilt.

You don't feel worthy of peace, so you reject it.
You don't believe you deserve good things, so you sabotage them.
You think you're being noble by carrying the weight, but really you're just slowing yourself down.
It's not redemption - it's self-sabotage with a halo on it.

You Can't Hate Yourself Into a Version You Love.

No one ever healed from self-loathing.
You can't fix yourself with the same tools that broke you.
All that mental flogging?
The harsh inner dialogue, the way you replay every mistake, the punishment routines you call 'discipline'?
It's not making you better.
It's keeping you small.
Because self-respect isn't born out of suffering.
It's built through consistent action.
Not perfect action.
Not loud action.
Consistent, honest action.
You don't need to suffer more.
You need to forgive yourself and move with purpose.

Growth Without Forgiveness Is a House Built on Sand.

You can grind, hustle, and tick every damn box on the self-help checklist.
But if deep down, you're still running on the belief that you're broken, useless, or unworthy...
You'll find a way to make it all collapse.

You'll cower when success shows up.
You'll ghost your breakthrough.
You'll pull the pin on your progress and call it fate.
Why?
Because you're still operating on old code.
Guilt.
Shame.
Fear disguised as drive.

You haven't cleared your emotional malware.
Until you deal with your guilt, your shame, your past - you'll never trust your wins.
You'll think every success is a fluke.
Every good moment is borrowed.
And every stumble will whisper - *"See? I knew you'd fuck it up again."*

Put the Weapon Down.

Forgiveness isn't letting yourself off the hook.
It's acknowledging the hit, owning the lesson, and walking forward without dragging the corpse.
You don't owe your past a lifetime of misery.
You're not chained to your worst chapter unless you keep rereading it.
Let go.
You made the mistake.
You faced the consequence.
Now you make the change.
You don't have to keep bleeding just to prove it mattered.

The Real Work Is Grace, Not Grind.

You think you need another 5 a.m. start?
Another cold shower?
Another round of punishment dressed as self-improvement?
Maybe.

But maybe what you really need is to look yourself in the mirror and say -
"That's enough. I forgive you. Now let's fucking go."

You can't heal if you're still holding the knife.
You can't grow if you're still punishing the version of you that didn't know better.
And you can't lead, love, or win if you keep dragging shame into every new arena you step into.

So cut the cord.
Drop the guilt.
Put the weapon down.
And finally let yourself run.

Put It On the Table.

Does this 'thought' hit home?
☐ Yes   ☐ Not really

If yes, can you call yourself out and apply it?
☐ Yes   ☐ Still hiding

If yes, what's one move you'll make to prove it's not just words?

....

....

Thought 8
Progress Looks Like Chaos Before It Looks Like Clarity.

Everyone wants to change.
No one wants the mess that comes with it.
You set out to improve your body, mindset, business, relationship -
and suddenly it feels like you're juggling flaming knives while
blindfolded on a skateboard in the dark.
Naked.

Shit breaks.
You forget things.
You snap at people you love.
You look in the mirror and think, *"Am I actually getting worse?"*
Maybe.
And maybe that's exactly what's supposed to happen.
Because that's what progress looks like.
At least in the beginning.

Change Destroys Before It Builds.

Growth isn't clean.
It's not a sunrise yoga montage.
It's demolition.
You can't build a cathedral without tearing down what stood there
before.

Old habits, weak beliefs, soft routines - they don't go quietly.
They scream.
They dig their claws in.
They beg to stay.

So when you decide to level up, expect rubble.
Your routines will feel off.
You'll sleep worse before you sleep better.
You'll question your plan, your identity, your worth.
You'll feel awkward, out of sync, clumsy, emotional.
That's not a red flag.
That's the cost of construction.
It's not a glow-up.
It's a grind-up.
And it's messy as hell before it ever looks magical.

People Mistake Turbulence for a Sign to Quit.

Here's where most people bail.
They think the confusion, the wobble, the second-guessing is a sign
they're not cut out for it.
Nah mate - that's just turbulence.
The plane's still climbing.

Everyone's obsessed with 'alignment' and 'flow'.
Everyone's waiting for the perfect vibe, the green light from the
universe, the clean emotional runway.
But real alignment?
Sometimes it only shows up after.
After you've dragged yourself through a war zone.
That's when things start to click.

Everyone posts the after photo.
No one posts the part where they're bloated, anxious, and screaming
at the NutriBullet because they can't twist the fucking lid off.
Progress doesn't announce itself with trumpets.

It arrives dressed as confusion, self-doubt, and a 5 a.m. identity crisis in a cold bathroom mirror.

You're Supposed to Feel Lost.

There is no map for reinvention.
No blueprint for becoming someone you've never been before.
You are building a version of yourself from the ground up.
Of course it feels shaky.
Of course you're doubting everything.
You're leaving a life you knew for a future that doesn't even exist yet.
The sooner you stop expecting growth to feel like a motivational reel and start accepting it might feel like a nervous breakdown, the sooner you'll move.

The Ugly Phase Is Sacred.

You know that middle part of a haircut where it looks like shit?
The awkward in-between phase?
That's where most people panic and shave it all off again.
Same thing with growth.
There's a sacred window in every transformation where everything looks and feels worse before it gets better.
Your confidence drops.
Your habits haven't stuck yet.
The new identity doesn't quite fit, and the old one's already dead.
Welcome to the halfway headfuck.
The womb of transformation.
Stay there.
Don't abort the mission just because it's messy.

Discomfort Is a Signpost, Not a Stop Sign.

Discomfort isn't danger.
It's the death rattle of your old life.

When you start choosing effort over ease, your nervous system flinches.
When you say "*no*" where you used to say "*yes*", people squirm.
When you raise your standards, your comfort zone starts a riot.
That resistance?
That stretch between who you were and who you're becoming?
That's not chaos.
That's calibration.
It's your nervous system learning it doesn't have to panic when you act with power.
It's your brain learning it can survive without approval.
It's your habits learning they don't own you anymore.
The noise is a good sign.
It means the old pattern knows its time is up.

Most People Quit in the Gap.

More often than not, there's a time lag between the reps and the results.
Sometimes it's days.
Sometimes months.
Sometimes it feels like you're giving everything and getting fuck-all back.
And in that gap?
Your doubt gets loud.
Your excuses get clever.
Your willpower gets tested like it owes the universe money.

I quit smoking 15 years ago.
Day one, a single figure appeared on my shoulder.
Sharp suit, yellow fingers, smirking.
He whispered, "*Smoke, smoke, smoke,*" like a cursed lullaby.
On day two, he brought backup.
Day three, more arrived.
Little soldiers of death, marching from shoulder to shoulder, drilling their orders into my skull, "*Smoke, smoke, SMOKE!*"

By the end of week one, dozens of the little fuckers were threading themselves through my nervous system, short-circuiting my focus, rewiring my patience, pulling the strings of my emotions like sadistic puppeteers.
By week four, they were everywhere.
A full-blown invasion.
Hundreds of the miniature tyrants of death, in formation, barking doubt into every crack of willpower they could find.
And then…
Silence.
Not all at once.
But one by one, they started to vanish.
Quietly.
Without a fight.
Like cowards who realised I wasn't folding.
Two months in, they were gone.
And I was free from my nicotine-plated tormentors.

That's what the gap feels like.
You're not just resisting temptation, you're battling an army.
And that army only retreats when it knows you won't surrender.
Most people don't last that long.
They mistake the noise for truth.
Don't make that mistake.
The chaos is a signal.
The resistance is proof you're close.

Stop Looking for Perfect. Start Looking for Proof.

Perfect doesn't exist.
It's a mirage - a shiny lie that stalls momentum and kills progress.
Perfect is the drug that keeps you dreaming instead of doing.
You chase the perfect time, perfect body, perfect plan, instead of proof.
And while you're waiting for stars to align, someone else is out there stacking proof.

So, ditch perfect.
Start looking for evidence.
Did you do one uncomfortable thing today?
Did you honour a new standard instead of defaulting to old habits?
Did you show up even a little when it would've been easier to bail?
That's what matters.
That's what stacks.
That's what compounds into clarity.

Be Proud of the Mess.

So next time you're knee-deep in the mess - overwhelmed and
exhausted - wondering if you're fucking it all up...
Pause.
Breathe.
And remember this -
Progress looks like chaos before it looks like clarity.
If it's ugly, it means you're in motion.
If it's noisy, it means something's shifting.
If it's scary, it means you're alive.
Don't back off.
Lean in.
Because one day you'll wake up in the clarity.
Not because you waited.
Not because the universe gifted it to you.
But because you built it.
Brick by messy, uncertain, unglamorous brick.

Put It On the Table.

Does this 'thought' hit home?
☐ Yes   ☐ Not really

If yes, can you call yourself out and apply it?
☐ Yes   ☐ Still hiding

If yes, what's one move you'll make to prove it's not just words?

....

....

Thought 9
Resentment Is Just Unexpressed Cowardice.

Y ou didn't speak up.
Now you're bitter.
That's on you.
Resentment doesn't make you righteous.
It makes you a mute lemon.
Silent and sour.
You weren't walked on, you laid down.
You weren't overlooked, you kept your mouth shut.
You weren't betrayed, you watched the line get crossed and stood still.
That's not strength.
That's self-abandonment in a polished mask.

Silence Isn't Noble. It's Convenient.

Most people confuse silence with maturity.
They call it 'rising above.'
But it's not enlightenment.
It's avoidance with lipstick.
You were scared.
Scared of confrontation.
Scared of being 'too much'.
Scared someone might label you needy, or difficult, or dramatic.
So you played the part.
Smiled.
Nodded.

Shrunk.
Now you're not mad at them.
You're pissed off at yourself.
Because deep down, you know - you trained them to treat you this way.

Resentment Is the Invoice for Your Cowardice.

It doesn't arrive right away.
It shows up later, quietly, but with interest.
The discomfort you ducked back then?
It's now a burning knot in your chest.
You said *"yes"* when your whole body was screaming *"no."*
You kept making room for people who never even noticed your bleeding
feet.
And now?
You're pacing the kitchen.
Clenching your jaw.
Rerunning the scene like a courtroom drama in your head.
Still not saying the thing.
Still choosing quiet over clarity.
Still swallowing your truth like it's noble.
It's not.
It's just easier.
And you're choking on it.

Being 'Easygoing' Isn't a Personality - It's a Disguise.

You think being agreeable makes you lovable.
You think if you're nice enough, quiet enough, helpful enough - no one will ever leave you.
They will.
People-pleasers don't get loyalty.
They get used.

And underneath all that 'flexibility'?
Is fear.
Fear of being too much.
Fear of being disliked.
Fear of being told, *"You're the only one who had a problem."*
You're not generous.
You're terrified.
And if you keep pretending otherwise, the resentment will rot you from the inside out.

Your Mouth Is Closed, Your Rage Is Loud.

Every time you bite your tongue, you pay for it later.
Every *"it's fine"* when it's not.
Every moment you fake agreement to avoid the sting of honesty.
Brick by brick, you build a wall around yourself.
Until it caves in.
Want to stop resenting them?
Say the thing.
Not when it's safe.
When it matters.
Not to your friend, your group chat, or your journal - to them.
Directly.
Calmly.
Early.

You Don't Get to Complain About What You Tolerate.

If you won't confront it - you co-sign it.
You're not just a victim - you're a co-author.
By saying nothing, you said, *"This is acceptable."*
And now you're stuck in a script you helped write - one where your needs don't matter.
One where your silence became the plot.
Don't like the story?
Change the damn plot.

Rock the Boat or Sink With It.

The world teaches you to stay smooth.
"*Keep the peace.*"
"*Don't make a scene.*"
"*Be the bigger person.*"
But what if the peace is fake?
What if the cost of keeping everyone else comfortable is slowly erasing yourself?
Sometimes the boat needs to be rocked.
Sometimes being the bigger person means planting your feet and saying, "*No. That's not okay with me.*"
You don't need to scream.
You don't need to shake.
You just need to mean it.

Silence Isn't Neutral - It's Destructive.

Unspoken resentment doesn't disappear.
It metastasises.
It twists your perception.
It stains every conversation.
It turns you into someone bitter, brittle, and passive-aggressive.
You think you're being patient?
You're rotting.
If you never say what matters, don't act shocked when it doesn't get respected.
People respond to the boundaries you enforce, not the ones you hope they notice.
You're not here to train the world to decode your sighs.
You're here to tell the truth.
Out loud.
To their face.
Without a smirk or a side-eye or a three-week delay.

I Froze, I Failed, I Remember.

I was at uni, living in a shared house with a fat bloke called Luke, and
a cockney called Chris with fucking dreadful teeth.
One night, we all went out.
Luke pulled a girl and brought her home.
The next morning, she was still asleep upstairs.
Luke was in the kitchen bragging.
Loud.
Crude.
Graphic.
Chris egged him on - two idiots gloating like they'd just won a trophy.
Then it got worse.
They started messing with her stuff.
Ripped the heels off her shoes.
Filled her handbag with ketchup.
And shoved her phone somewhere I won't repeat.
And I just sat there.
Frozen.
Button-bashing FIFA '06 while they humiliated her in absence.
Something in me twisted.
I wanted to speak.
I wanted to shout.
I wanted to throw them both through the fucking wall.
But I didn't.
I stayed quiet.
Told myself it wasn't my business.
Told myself she wouldn't find out.
Told myself it wasn't that bad.
Lies.
All of it.
Because she did find out.
She came downstairs an hour later, holding her bag like it was a dead
thing.
Tears in her eyes.
No words.
Just shame.
Thick, silent, and heavy enough to choke the room.

She left.
And we all just carried on.

That silence has lived inside me for eighteen years.
I've done a lot since.
Got stronger.
Sharper.
Louder.
But that moment lives in my bones.
The way I froze.
The way I let fear beat out integrity.
The way I let someone get hurt because I didn't want the conflict.

People treat regrets like rare coins.
I think most of us are carrying a few that never go away.
They live just under the surface.
Waiting for quiet moments to remind you who you were - and who you weren't.
No - I wasn't the villain in that story.
But I wasn't the man I wanted to be either.
I was there.
I saw it.
And I said nothing.
And that silence?
Cost more than any punch ever could.

Bitterness Is Just Honesty You Were Too Afraid to Voice.

If you're bitter, check your silence.
Ask yourself - where did I shrink?
Where did I trade honesty for harmony?
Where did I let politeness dig my grave?
Because bitterness is just backed-up bravery.
Courage you left on the shelf when it counted.
The words you swallowed until they soured.
So, use it now.
Say the thing.

Set the boundary.
Speak the line.
Even if your voice shakes.
You don't have to scream - you just have to stop pretending you're fine.

Put It On the Table.

Does this 'thought' hit home?
☐ Yes ☐ Not really

If yes, can you call yourself out and apply it?
☐ Yes ☐ Still hiding

If yes, what's one move you'll make to prove it's not just words?

....

....

Part 2

BUILD THE FIRE

Thought 10
Scars > Filters.

Skip the highlight reels.
Forget curated chaos.
Ditch the captions masking collapse.
Let's talk about the truth.
The wreckage.
The rebuilds.
The scar tissue that doesn't show in photos.
The kind of pain that rewires you.
The kind of growth that doesn't even look like growth until years later.
Because here's the unvarnished reality...
Scars beat filters.
Every time.

Filters Conceal, Scars Reveal.

A filter's easy.
Swipe.
Crop.
Caption.
Throw a nice preset over the clusterfuck and call it 'clarity'.
It's performative.
Tidy.
Controlled.
A romanticised disaster.
We clean up the chaos for the camera.
Highlight the comeback, blur the breakdown.
Package the pain so it looks poetic instead of real.

But a scar?
A scar is messy and earned.
It costs something.
A scar means you didn't just experience pain.
You survived it.
It's what's left after the bleeding stops.
Not decorative.
Definitive.

A filter says, "*look at me!*"
A scar says, "*I'm still here.*"
A filter wonders, "*Do I look okay?*"
A scar declares, "*I made it through what should've ended me.*"
Filters seek approval.
Scars tell the truth.

Through Fire, Not Around It.

I'm an addict.
Not was.
Am.
Drink, drugs and full throttle chaos.
That was my diet for years.
And I'm not wrapping it in metaphors or softening it for comfort.
It nearly killed me.
But it didn't.

And twenty years sober later, it's still a daily fight.
Not a one-time decision.
Not a finish line you cross.
It's a relentless commitment.
A decision I remake every day.
It's choosing to feel what I once numbed.
Choosing presence when dissociation would be easier.
Choosing to hurt cleanly.

People love a recovery story.
The polished before-and-after montage.
But the middle?
The thousand quiet battles?
No one applauds that part.
But that's where everything changed.
My eyes didn't just clear, they evolved.
My scar didn't just close, it rewired me.
Made me more patient.
More dangerous.
More human.
I see the underdog and never underestimate them.
I back the black sheep.
Stand with the broken.
Because I've been them.
I know what it costs to stay.
To rebuild.
To rise without applause.
I'm smarter now.
And none of that wisdom came from a filter.
It came from fire.
From clawing through chaos with bare hands.
From a scar.

Lead With Your Scar.

There's power in not hiding.
In walking into a room and refusing to perform.
Not reshaping your story to make it easier to swallow.
Not shrinking your truth just to keep the peace.
Just... showing up.
Scar out.
Shoulders back.
Unapologetic.
Because when you stop hiding, you create space.
And people feel it.

They feel the difference between someone who's polished, and someone who's whole.

When you lead with your scar, you tell the room, *"It's safe to be real here."*

You give people permission to put their armour down.
To stop pretending.
To finally admit what they've been holding in.

It's not about oversharing.
It's about standing in your story without shame.
And that?
That's magnetic.
It doesn't draw people to your strength.
It draws them to your sincerity.
Your scar becomes the safest place in the room.
Not because it's neat or resolved, but because it's true.
And truth?
It's what we're all dying for - beneath the filters and the scripts and the smiles that don't reach the eyes.
So lead with your scar.
Not because it defines you, but because it reminds the rest of us we're not alone.

To the Ones Still Hiding

I see you.
Still pretending it doesn't hurt.
Still curating your collapse to make it look like strength.
Still terrified someone might see the real you.
Let me tell you something -
Your cracks aren't the danger.
Your silence is.
Let people in.
Not everyone. Not all at once.
But someone.
Let them see the scars.
Let them hear the unfiltered version.

The version that didn't win.
The version that barely made it.
You don't owe anyone perfection.
You owe yourself honesty.
Scars don't make you weak.
They make you unmistakable.
They mean you've crawled through fire and come back not empty-handed, but with wisdom.
With grit.
With a voice that no longer shakes when it speaks the truth.
So stop shrinking.
Stop hiding.
Start owning what you've earned.
Because that scar?
That's your crown.

Put It On the Table.

Does this 'thought' hit home?
☐ Yes   ☐ Not really

If yes, can you call yourself out and apply it?
☐ Yes   ☐ Still hiding

If yes, what's one move you'll make to prove it's not just words?

....

....

Thought 11
The Anatomy of the Relentless.

Y ou can put people into buckets -
People who coast.
People who grind.
People who talk.
People who move.
People who love the idea of better, until it requires actual effort.
And then there's a different breed entirely…
PB chasers.

Not your 'rise and grind' dopamine junkies.
Not the hashtag warriors or performative hustlers.
I'm talking about the ones who are quietly and methodically trying to
outwork yesterday's version of themselves.
No spotlight.
No shortcuts.
Just pure, unfiltered war with their own limits.
Those people?
Fear them.
Because if they can suffer on purpose, without applause, imagine
what else they can do when it counts.

I Got a New PB.

Marathon.
3 hours, 43 minutes, 7 seconds.
Yeah, the crowd was there.

The roar was real.
But the real victory?
That happened long before I tied my laces.
It happened because I trained when it was boring.
When it hurt.
When I didn't feel like it.
Because PBs don't come to people who dabble.
They come to people who decide - no ifs, ands, or buts.

Here's what most people get wrong...
Chasing a PB isn't just about the stopwatch - it's about the mentality.
You're not just trying to move faster - you're trying to become
someone who doesn't flinch when the inner demons get rowdy and
the pain hits.

Training Is the Test.

Most people train like they're waiting to be motivated.
PB chasers?
They train like the outcome's already written - they just have to earn it.
It's not glamorous.
It's not sexy.
It's weeks of frozen hands on early runs, missed social plans and
tracking macronutrients like it's a religion.
Reviewing splits, cadence, and stride length.
Doing rehab for injuries that haven't even happened yet - just in case.
That's not grind - that's discipline without a pat on the head.

PB chasers don't chase hype - they hunt the hard gains.
Because they know something most people don't...
You don't get the life you want.
You get the one you trained for.

Race Day Is the Real You, Uncensored.

Here's the myth - race day is where it all happens.

Here's the truth - race day reveals what you built in private.
Nothing more.
Nothing less.
It magnifies every shortcut you took.
Every session you skipped.
Every excuse you called reasonable.
On that day?
There's nowhere to hide.
Soft doubts soon scream.
Pain shows up with receipts.
And the work you did - or didn't do - stays beside you every mile.

And when that happens, the fakes fall apart.
The real ones?
They lean in.
They're not shocked by the pain.
They trained for it.
They're not overwhelmed by the distance.
They respected it.
They don't need hype music or cheering crowds.
Their grit is internal.
The butterflies of nerves don't flutter anymore - they salute and fall in line.

The Three Stages of the Inner War.

Stage 1 : Discipline.
The first third.
You feel good.
Almost too good.
That's the trap.
Your ego fires the starting gun - *"Let's fucking go!"*
But your training whispers - *"Stick to the plan."*
And right there is the first battle - deny the ego.
Obey the blueprint.

It's not about pace.
It's about patience.

Stage 2 : Focus.
The middle miles.
No more buzz.
No real pain yet.
Just you, the road, and the rhythm.
Breath.
Cadence.
Posture.
Presence.
This is the zone where mastery lives - quiet, steady, earned.
Thousands of invisible reps paying off in silence.
No drama.
No crowd.
Just calm repetition and honest effort.
This is where the untrained drift.
This is where the prepared click in.

Stage 3 : Suffering.
The last third.
My favourite.
The body's not whispering anymore - it's screaming.
Quads burning.
Chest pounding.
Ankles aching.
Every step is a negotiation.
Every breath asks the same question, *"Why the fuck are you still doing this?"*
And from somewhere deep - somewhere primal - a voice answers.
Not loud.
Not poetic.
Just two words…
"Keep going."

That voice isn't motivational.
It's savage.

It's feral.
It lives for this.
You don't get it from books or mantras.
You build it.
By suffering on purpose.
By chasing PBs through hell and smiling anyway.

The Finish Line Is a Funeral for Old Limits.

When you cross, there's no fireworks.
Just inner peace.
A sacred moment of stillness where you realise you are not who you were when you started.
That version of you - the one who couldn't do this?
You buried them on the course.
They died somewhere in the middle miles.
Under the weight of your grit.
Under 42 km of pain, doubt, and relentless forward motion.
That's why PB chasers walk differently.
Not because they're arrogant - because they've seen their own edge, and kept going anyway.

The Ceiling Gets Closer. The Fight Gets Dirtier.

Here's the kicker -
Each PB gets harder.
You're no longer shaving minutes - you're chasing seconds.
Tiny, brutal gains - millimetres of progress earned with miles of pain.
And there's no guarantee you'll get it.
You might give your all and still fall short.
But that's what makes it worth it.
PB chasers don't chase ease.
They chase the edge.
And every time they reach it, they sharpen it.

That mindset bleeds into everything -

Into business.
Into art.
Into parenting.
Into relationships.
You start showing up differently.
Because once you've learned how to suffer for progress - mediocrity starts to taste like ash.

PB Chasers Don't Wait to Feel Like It.

They don't check the weather.
They don't ask their feelings for permission.
They don't wait for motivation to knock.
They run in storms.
They lift when they're tired.
They show up on the days they'd rather disappear.

Because the goal isn't to feel great - the goal is to be undeniable.
That's what makes them dangerous.
They don't need permission.
They don't chase applause.
They don't post about it.
They've got their own scoreboard - and they update it daily.

Respect the Relentless.

If you've got someone in your life chasing PBs - don't mock it.
Don't downplay it.
Don't roll your eyes and say, *"It's just running"* or *"You're taking it too seriously."*
What they're doing isn't about sport.
It's about proving they can become someone they weren't before.
That kind of hunger doesn't shut off when the race ends.
That kind of fire lives in their bones.

So if you see someone quietly chasing a new version of themselves...

Step back.
Or level up.
Because PB chasers don't stop.
They just raise the bar.
Again.
And again.
And again.

Put It On the Table.

Does this 'thought' hit home?
☐ Yes   ☐ Not really

If yes, can you call yourself out and apply it?
☐ Yes   ☐ Still hiding

If yes, what's one move you'll make to prove it's not just words?

....

....

Thought 12
Busy Bullshit.

L et's stop pretending.
 "I don't have time" is just adult code for *"I can't be fucked."*
It's a get-out-of-jail-free card we throw down to dodge responsibility.
You weren't too busy.
You just chose something else.
Something easier.
Safer.
Softer.
And that's okay - just call it what it is.
Because every time you say, *"I don't have time,"* what you're really saying is, *"It wasn't a priority."*

Time Isn't the Problem. Priorities Are.

You had time to doomscroll until your thumb cramped.
You had time to rewatch *'The Office'* *"for background noise"* - again.
You had time to chase validation, argue with strangers, and refresh your feed like your life depended on it.
But carve out 30 minutes for something that actually matters?
Suddenly you're swamped.

It's not about minutes.
It's about meaning.
You weren't short on time.
You were short on fire.
If it mattered, you'd already be moving.
You wouldn't be waiting for motivation to give you permission.
You'd show up.

Relentlessly.

Tired? Go.
Doubtful? Go.
Confused? Go anyway.
Because when something burns in your chest, you don't find time -
you protect it.
You carve it from bone.
You cut the fluff, the noise, the nonsense.
And that takes guts.
It takes confronting the brutal truth - most people stay busy to avoid
admitting they're not committed.

Busy Is Just a Costume.

Everyone's busy.
Everyone's tired.
Everyone's juggling bills, kids, deadlines, and drama.
But some people use that weight to fuel a mission.
Others wear it like a mask.

You think your life is uniquely complicated?
You think you've got a monopoly on stress?
You don't.
There's a single parent out there working two jobs and still building a
business on their lunch break.
There's a kid with no savings starting something on a cracked phone
from a library's Wi-Fi connection.
Time is neutral.
What you do with it?
That's where character shows up.

Productivity vs. Performance.

Here's the trap - confusing motion with meaning.
Mistaking a full calendar for a full life.

Wearing, *"I've got so much on"* - like a personality.
You fill your day with checklists, dashboards, back-to-back calls.
Tasks that nibble at the edges of importance, but never touch the centre.
You clear your inbox.
You schedule calls.
You update spreadsheets, optimise systems, and answer every fucking
Slack notification within 30 seconds like it's a test of character.
And yeah, it looks like you're on fire.
But inside?
You're stuck.

Because productivity is not performance.
Productivity is doing a lot.
Performance is doing what matters.
And most people will do absolutely anything to avoid the work that actually counts.
Why?
Because high performance demands exposure.
It asks you to bring your edge.
It risks judgement.
It forces you to show up in arenas where effort isn't enough - you need courage, clarity, and consequences.
It's easy to get good at being busy.
It's hard to sit down and build something that might not work.
To say, *"This is what I really want"* - and then move like you mean it.
So instead?
You stay useful, but never vulnerable.
You stay in motion, but never create momentum.
You work around the edge of your purpose, but never through the middle.
And slowly, silently, you become excellent at everything...
Except the thing that matters.

Time Freedom Is a Myth.

Everyone fantasises about time freedom.
"If I just had a few free days."
"If I didn't have this job."
"If I could just get a break…"
Here's the harsh truth - if you're not making use of the scraps of time you do have, you won't know what to do with the whole damn banquet.
You'd waste it.
You'd sleep more.
Scroll more.
Complain more.
Discipline isn't born when life gives you space.
It's born when you take space - right in the middle of the chaos.

People Will Understand When You're Dead.

Everyone wants to be understood.
But if that's your main driver?
You're already cooked.
People don't 'get it' until you've done it.
Only when the thing is finished do the missed calls, locked doors, late nights, quiet exits suddenly make sense.
Until then?
"You've changed."
"You're selfish."
"You're too intense."
Let them talk.
The ones who finish?
They've made peace with being misunderstood.
They don't explain.
They don't defend.
They don't justify.
They build. Quietly.
Obsessively.
Unapologetically.

And the applause shows up at the funeral, when the mission's already complete.

The Time Audit Test.

Want to see the truth?
Audit your last 72 hours.
Track every minute.
Brutally.
Now ask yourself - how much went to things that matter?
How much to comfort?
How much to other people's drama?
Now ask yourself - if someone else had to read this schedule out loud as your obituary - would you be proud?
If the answer's *"hell no"* - change it.

The Time Compass.

Most people don't need more time, they need a working Time Compass.
I've capitalised the first letters of 'Time Compass' as if it's a known thing - it's not.
I've made it up.
A Time Compass is something that doesn't just track hours, but points you toward what actually matters.
And the truth is most people's compass is fucked.
It spins like a drunk sailor.
Pulled by dopamine.
Hijacked by distractions.
Warped by fake urgency and the pressure to perform for people they don't even fucking like.
So they end up busy but not purposeful.
Active but not aligned.
You want clarity?
Stop staring at the clock and ask yourself - *"Where's my true north?"*
"What actually moves the needle?"

"What's worth bleeding for?"
Once you find that?
Time stops being the problem.
The noise dies down.
The bullshit gets filtered out.
When your compass is fixed, everything else starts to follow.

Steal Time Back.

You don't need more hours.
You need boundaries with teeth.
Here's where to start…
Wake up before your excuses.
Stop checking your phone like it holds the answer.
Say *"no"* like it's a prayer.
Book your dream like it's a job interview.
Show up when it's boring.
Especially when it's boring.
Because doing it badly still gets you further than waiting to do it
perfectly.
And showing up messy still crushes the version of you who never
starts.

Stop Lying in the Gap.

You're either in or you're not.
No more pretending.
No more half-arsed *"maybe next week"* plans.
Own your choices.
If you want it - go get it.
If you don't - shut the fuck up about it.
But don't sit in the middle lane, blinking your indicator for a life you've
got no real intention of turning into.
You're not too busy.
You're just not ready.
Yet.

Put It On the Table.

Does this 'thought' hit home?
☐ Yes   ☐ Not really

If yes, can you call yourself out and apply it?
☐ Yes   ☐ Still hiding

If yes, what's one move you'll make to prove it's not just words?

....

....

Thought 13
Execution Eats Insight.

We're drowning in content and starving for action.
You've got more tools, tactics, and 'how-tos' at your fingertips than any generation in history.
Want to build a brand?
Lose weight?
Get rich?
Heal trauma?
Write a book?
Become a fucking monk?
It's all there - one click away.
And still, most are frozen.
Scrolling.
Consuming.
Doing fuck all.
Because the problem was never access.
The problem is execution.

If you're always learning but never building, you're not progressing.
You're hoarding.
And hoarding isn't growth - it's stagnation dressed up as productivity.

You're Not Learning, You're Collecting.

Every time you highlight a quote in a book, double-tap a carousel post, or nod along to a podcast and then do nothing with it - you're training your brain to confuse insight with impact.
Let that sink in.

You don't need a new strategy - you need to honour the one already sitting in your notes app.

Reading five books on leadership won't make you a leader.
Ten episodes on habit change won't make you disciplined.
You already know that.
But collection feels good - it gives you a hit of momentum without any risk.
A hit of forward motion without demanding skin in the game.
That's the trap.
Collection is painless - it feels good without risk.
It lets you fantasise about potential without facing resistance.
But here's the truth…
If your knowledge doesn't make it to your calendar, your reps, your actions - it's not real.
It's just noise in the system.

Input Without Output Creates Paralysis.

Too much input and not enough output creates confusion.
Paralysis by possibility.
You've consumed so many perspectives that you've stopped trusting your own.
You've over-analysed every option until every step feels wrong.
So you freeze.
You tell yourself -
"I just need more clarity."
"One more podcast."
"Another coffee with a mentor."
But clarity doesn't come from knowing everything - it comes from choosing something and moving.
And only in motion do the answers start showing up.

Intellectual Hoarding Is Just Fear in Fancy Clothes.

What you're doing isn't prep.

It's avoidance.
You're scared.
Scared of looking stupid.
Scared of starting messy.
Scared of being seen trying and still falling short.
So instead, you hide behind research.
You cloak your fear in, "*I'm just learning.*"
You talk like a guru but live like a ghost.
That makes you smart…
But not dangerous.
The ones who actually shift things?
Who move culture, build communities, launch ideas?
They're not sitting on 100 highlighted quotes.
They're publishing their 10th imperfect post.
They're not collecting - they're compounding.

Overconsumption Makes You Passive.

There's a reason most content feels like junk food.
It's engineered to keep you scrolling, watching, nodding - but never moving.
You've been trained to consume, not create.
To feel fired up by other people's actions instead of taking your own.

And slowly, passively, you become an expert on journeys you've never taken.
You quote the greats.
You bookmark the advice.
You nod along like a disciple at the Church of Progress.
But when it's your turn to move?
Crickets.
You watch others live out your ambitions from the comfort of your curated feed.
That's not education - it's entertainment dressed up in personal growth packaging.

Build or Be Forgotten.

You want to matter?
Make something.
You want to stand out?
Finish something that scares you.
You want to grow?
Create friction.
Put your name on something that can be critiqued, broken, improved.

The people you admire?
They're not smarter than you.
They're just louder with their actions.
They've hit publish.
They've launched.
They've been wrong - and kept going anyway.

You don't become a writer by reading.
You become a writer by writing.
You don't become a creator by learning platforms.
You become one by uploading that first messy draft.
You don't become a leader by reading - *'The Diary Of A CEO'*.
You become one by having the hard conversation no one else will.

Action Is a Muscle. Train It.

Every day you delay output, that muscle atrophies.
Every time you hesitate, it gets harder to move.
And you're either training it, or letting it wither.
Every pause feeds the paralysis.
Every excuse becomes a brick in the wall you'll have to punch through later.
So start small.
Say the thing you've been rehearsing in your head for months.
Write the ugly draft.
Record the shaky voice note.
Pitch the offer.

Make a mess.
Make noise.
Fall on your face if you have to.
Because while you're overthinking, someone else is overtaking.
And by the time you finally feel 'ready', the opportunity's already moved
on - and so has your competition.

Output doesn't just create results, it creates momentum.
It builds self-trust.
It teaches you how to adjust in real-time, rather than waiting for a plan
to be perfect (which it never will be).

Turn Input into Ammunition.

Here's the upgrade…
Every time you learn something new, ask yourself -
"What can I apply from this in the next 24 hours?"
"What decision does this help me make?"
"What action does this clarify?"
If the answer is nothing?
Bin it.
If it's useful?
Move.
Input becomes powerful the moment it leads to a decision.
Otherwise, it's just self-help masturbation.

Forget Perfection. Chase Progress.

Stop waiting to be ready.
You're not here to be perfect - you're here to progress.
That means fumbling the first reps.
That means building in public - even when it's messy.
That means jumping in before the confidence shows up.
You want to feel alive again?

Stop playing mental Jenga with your ideas and start using your fucking hands.
Make noise that matters.
Write the blog.
Post the video.
Send the pitch.
Design the thing.

Your value isn't in what you know - it's in what you build.
Your portfolio isn't your thoughts - it's your trail of proof.
Every output is a vote for who you're becoming - so start casting votes.

What Did You Do This Week?

Not what you bookmarked.
Not what you highlighted.
Not what you journaled about or spoke to your coach about.
What did you build?
A brick in your business?
A post that scared you?
A workout that pushed your edge?
A piece of work that made you sweat?

If the answer is nothing... then all that input was just noise.
You weren't downloading insights.
You were distracting yourself from execution.

Put It On the Table.

Does this 'thought' hit home?
☐ Yes   ☐ Not really

If yes, can you call yourself out and apply it?
☐ Yes   ☐ Still hiding

If yes, what's one move you'll make to prove it's not just words?

....

....

Thought 14
Put Up or Shut Up.

There's a type of person that makes my knuckles twitch.
They show up, strike a pose, go through the motions - perfect posture, zero pressure.
Squatting air, calling it effort.
Hiding their cowardice behind hashtags and dead men's words.
They want the look of discipline without the cost.
That's not training.
That's self-delusion with a soundtrack.
No discomfort?
No growth.
No pain?
No point.
No sacrifice?
No progress.

No Strain, No Gain.

You can have the cleanest plan, the freshest gear, the boldest quote tattooed on your forearm.
None of it matters.
If there's no resistance, you're just shadowboxing your potential.
Real effort hurts.
It smells like sweat, panic, and persistence.
It's messy.
Quiet.
Repetitive.

It begins exactly where your comfort ends.
If it doesn't bruise your ego, it won't build you.
If it doesn't threaten your pride, it won't shift your limits.

Progress lives where excuses get loud.
Where your body barks, your mood nosedives, and your brain pleads,
"Skip it.
Do it tomorrow."
That's the gate.
And most people bow out.
They mistake struggle for danger.
But real ones?
They recognise it as the invitation.

You want to change?
You've got to risk failure.
Risk being seen.
Risk falling flat in front of people who expect you to quit.
Risk coming up short.
Because anything less is just performance.
Just reps without resistance.

The Race That Rewired Me.

Seventy kilometres into 'Race to the Stones' and I was fucked.
Proper fucked.
I was in the middle of a field, head torch on, being attacked by a gang
of giant moths.
Blisters blooming.
Stomach twisted.
Blood seeping through the toe-box of my white Nikes.
Everything screamed - tap out.
Lie down.
Vanish.
Then... Goggins.
Not the man (obvs), but the voice.
Echoing through my skull...

"When you think you're done, you're only at 40%."

I'd quoted it before.
Posted it.
But this time I heard it.
I didn't surge forward.
I didn't rally.
I just... refused to quit.
One step.
One breath.
Repeat.

I crossed the finish line just after 4am.
Chip time - 21 hours 14 minutes 06 seconds.
And a new mind inside my old body.

That race didn't just test my limits.
It reset them.
It taught me exhaustion is mostly negotiation.
And most people fold before the contract even hits the table.

Don't Say It. Carry It.

You want to prove something?
Don't talk - carry.
Plans, calendars, vision boards - they mean fuck all without load.
The effort you put in when no one's watching?
That's who you are.
That's the real résumé.
Don't show me your goals.
Show me the bruise behind your progress.
The burden behind your ambition.
The silence you've bled in, and kept showing up anyway.
Commitment isn't a vibe - it's a load-bearing truth.
No points for almost.
No medals for meaning to.
Just the bar.

The weight.
And your hands under it.
The bar doesn't give a fuck how tired you are.
Deadlines don't care how you feel.
You lift, or you don't.
Don't pose hungry if you're not gonna eat.

Training Hurts. That's the Point.

Most people aren't lazy.
They're just allergic to discomfort.
They'll work hard as long as it's easy.
But the second it stings - they flake.
The second it gets awkward, ugly, unglamorous - they bail.
No friction, no form.
No pressure, no progress.
If your training doesn't scare you a little, bore you a little, break you a little?..
It's not training.
It's pretending.
Sweatless and safe.

You Can't Fake Heavy.

You can fake busy.
You can fake hustle.
You can fake ambition.
But you can't fake heavy.
The weight doesn't care.
It doesn't respond to optics, only effort.
When things get heavy - whether it's responsibility, grief, pressure, or the bar - there's no pretending.
You lift… or you don't.
You hold… or you fold.
And if you fold?

That's not failure.
That's feedback.
That's the map to your current limit.
So now you've found the line.
Don't walk away from it.
Step up.
Get under it again.
And this time?
Start building past it.
That's where the real work begins.

The Grind You Can't See Still Bleeds.

It's easy to spot the grind in a gym -
The sweat.
The weight.
The repetition.
But what about the other kind?
The writer staring down a blinking cursor at 2 a.m.
The founder calculating payroll with two weeks of runway.
The artist tossing draft nine because it still isn't honest.
That's weight.
Unseen - but brutal.
Creating something from nothing doesn't just cost time.
It costs clarity.
It costs sanity.
It costs solitude.
No praise.
No finish line.
Just you and the terrifying freedom of the blank.

People say *"follow your passion"* like it's a picnic.
But passion fades.
Purpose doesn't.
And purpose?
It's heavy.
It demands more than most are willing to carry.

Because making something real means risking indifference.
It means bleeding truth onto the page or product - knowing most won't get it.
But you make it anyway.
Because not making it?
That's heavier.

The Bar Isn't Always Steel.

Sometimes the heaviest weight isn't on a rack.
Sometimes it's silence.
Sometimes it's a conversation you've been avoiding for years.
Sometimes it's standing behind your work when no one claps.
This isn't just about reps.
It's about the decision to carry.
To pick up what's yours - not because someone told you to, not because you're trying to impress the crowd, but because you know it's yours to lift.
Even when it's invisible to everyone else.
Even when it would be easier to drop it and walk the fuck away.

The Weight That Doesn't Show on the Scale.

It's in your parenting.
Your job.
Your relationships.
Your leadership.
Most think 'weight' means dumbbells and deadlifts.
But emotional reps?
They're often heavier.
Telling the truth when a lie is easier?
That's weight.
Asking for help when your pride is begging you to shut up?
That's weight.
Owning your flaws without collapsing into shame?
That's fucking heavy.

Vulnerability is resistance training for the soul.
It's not pretty. It doesn't get likes.
But it builds a spine that doesn't snap under pressure.
And just like physical training, most people ghost the second it burns.
They disappear.
Numb out.
Deflect.
Anything to avoid sitting in the discomfort.
But if your life is too light emotionally?
You're not building resilience - you're coasting in safety.
Want deeper love?
Say the hard thing.
Want real leadership?
Take heat you didn't cause.
Want peace?
Face chaos first.
So when I say "put weight on the bar," don't just think plates and reps.
Think truth under tension.
Think integrity when no one's watching.
Think emotional honesty under pressure.
Because growth isn't just strain - it's carrying what others never see,
bleeding in silence, and standing tall anyway.

Put It On the Table.

Does this 'thought' hit home?
☐ Yes   ☐ Not really

If yes, can you call yourself out and apply it?
☐ Yes   ☐ Still hiding

If yes, what's one move you'll make to prove it's not just words?

....

....

Thought 15
Multitasking Is a Myth.

It's a seductive lie we tell ourselves to feel accomplished while avoiding real depth.

You open fifteen tabs, juggle notifications, fire off emails while half-listening to a podcast, and convince yourself you're "*Getting shit done.*"

You're not.

Well... maybe you're getting shit done.

But it's just that.

Shit.

Low-quality, half-thought-through, scattered shit that leaves you drained and unsatisfied.

That isn't productivity.

It's a nervous habit dressed up as efficiency.

The Illusion of "Doing It All."

People love to say, "*I'm great at multitasking.*"

Translation - "*I'm used to living in constant distraction.*"

Real focus - the kind that builds things, solves problems, creates something meaningful - requires presence.

And presence doesn't split.

You either give your full mind to the moment or you give scraps.

Trying to do everything at once is the fastest way to do nothing that counts.

Busy Doesn't Equal Progress.

We treat 'busy' like some sort of badge of honour.
But 'busy' isn't brave.
It's often flustered avoidance.
You can be stacked with meetings, to-do lists, and inbox traffic and still and up exactly where you were six months ago.
Activity gives the illusion of progress while robbing you of real momentum.
True progress isn't loud or flashy.
It's usually slow.
Quiet.
Focused.
Less *"Look at me"* and more *"Fuck off and leave me alone, I'm building something."*

One Thing at a Time.

Want clarity?
Pick one thing.
Want power?
Protect that thing until it's done.
Multitasking might feel like control, but it's chaos wrapped in control's clothing.
The most effective people aren't jugglers.
They're choosers.
They choose their priority.
They honour it.
They finish it.
Then they move on.

Why Most People Feel Stuck.

Most people don't lack effort - they lack direction.
They're not lazy - they're leaking energy across too many fronts.
Scattered.

Pulled thin.
Drained by noon.
You start something… then -
Ping.
Scroll.
Ring.
Slack.
Zoom.
A partridge in a pear tree.
Gone.
Day's done.
You're fried.
And you're left wondering what actually moved forward.

It's not that you need to work harder.
You just need to focus better.

Attention Is Your Real Currency.

We treat time like it's the crown jewel - but it's not.
Attention is the currency.
And that's the resource you're bleeding out.
You could have a free afternoon, but if your brain's hooked on notification and alerts, you'll get jack shit done.
Every scroll, every click, every *"quick check"* takes a piece of your focus, and you can't reclaim it with caffeine or good intentions.
Your attention is sacred, and most people piss it away like it's nothing.

We chase stimulation as if it's purpose.
But it's not.
Stimulation is surface-level.
Progress lives in the deep waters.
Stillness?
That's where the good shit begins.
Awkward at first, sure - but it's the gateway.
Stay there.
That's where original thought lives.

Focus doesn't magically appear.
You have to design for it.
Close the tabs.
Silence the notifications.
Block the time.
And guard it like it's priceless.
Build a space where your mind can settle.
Because once it does - that's where the breakthroughs happen.

Mental Splinters.

Every time you context switch, every task half-started, every
conversation half-heard - you leave a splinter in your mind.
Tiny fragments of attention still hooked into tabs you forgot to close,
messages you half-replied to, decisions you didn't finish making.
They build up.
Like static.
Like clutter.
Like a thousand browser windows in your brain, all blinking for
attention.
By the end of the day, your brain becomes a cluttered room.
Lights on.
Drawers open.
Radio blasting three channels at once.
No wonder you're anxious.
No wonder you lie in bed exhausted but wired.
It's not the workload - it's the residue.
Mental inflammation from interruption after interruption.
But the real damage isn't just lost hours - it's what it does to your
inner world.

Because fragmented attention has a cost - and that cost is clarity.
It's creativity.
Presence.
Patience.
Peace.
When your focus is scattered, so is your identity.

You can't hear your intuition when everything's loud.
You can't go deep when you're constantly pulled to the surface.

You don't just do less.
You become less.
Less present.
Less rooted.
Less you.
And if you're not careful, that becomes your default.
A distracted life.
A diluted connection to yourself.
Reclaiming your attention isn't some productivity hack.
It's about finding your centre again.
You don't need a new routine.
You need to block out the noise and reconnect with yourself -
One breath.
One task.
One moment at a time.

Starter Finisher.

Most people ditch focus the moment they get bored.
But boredom is a sign you're close to something real.
It's the edge before immersion.
Stick with the task a little longer.
Go deeper.
What's on the other side isn't just productivity - it's pride.
The kind of pride that only comes from finishing something properly.
Forget the hack.
Forget the system.
Forget the planner.
Just finish something.
The thing you've been dancing around.
The task that keeps getting bumped down the list.
The uncomfortable, unsexy thing that actually matters.
Completion beats perfection.
Every time.

Because momentum doesn't come from thinking.
It comes from follow-through.

You don't need more hours in the day.
You need fewer distractions stealing the ones you already have.
Multitasking is comfort.
It's noise.
It's pretending.
Want to build something that matters?
Want to feel peace instead of pressure?
Pick what matters.
Show up fully.
Finish it well.

Because doing one thing right beats doing ten things at 10%.
Every.
Single.
Time.

Put It On the Table.

Does this 'thought' hit home?
☐ Yes   ☐ Not really

If yes, can you call yourself out and apply it?
☐ Yes   ☐ Still hiding

If yes, what's one move you'll make to prove it's not just words?

....

....

Thought 16
What You Do Daily Is Who You Are.

Your habits don't lie.
They just whisper the truth long after your mouth shuts up.
You can say all the right things, post the quotes, buy the planner, map out the dream.
But if your daily actions don't back it up, none of it means shit.
What you do on autopilot, in silence, when no one's watching - that's the real you.
Not your Sunday night promises.
Not your pumped-up podcast epiphanies.
The real you is found in the choices you make on a Tuesday morning when you're tired, distracted, and uninspired.
Your routine is either your ladder, or your leash.
And most people?
They're handcuffed to habits that quietly drag them in circles.

Proof Is in the Pattern.

You say you want growth.
A new level.
A sharper mindset.
But your habits suggest something else...
That you're more committed to comfort than change.
You wake up late.
Scroll Instagram before your feet touch the floor.
Eat like shit.

Avoid the hard stuff.
And call it, "*Just a phase.*"
It's not a phase.
It's a pattern.
And your patterns will always outvote your intentions.

If your morning starts in chaos, your mind will match it.
If your default is distraction, don't expect clarity.
If your actions are random, don't expect results.
You don't rise to your ambitions.
You fall to your rituals.
And your rituals are either weapons or weaknesses.

Start Ruthlessly Simple.

Change doesn't begin with some dramatic reset.
It starts with relentless repetition.
Not the sexy, cinematic stuff.
Just the non-negotiables that recalibrate your identity.
Get up when the alarm rings.
Water before caffeine.
Move your body before you move your thumbs.
Make one uncomfortable decision before breakfast.
Create something, anything, before consuming everything.

These aren't viral habits.
But they compound.
They don't just change your morning - they rewire who you believe
yourself to be.
And what they build is dangerous.
A version of you that doesn't wait for inspiration.
Doesn't need motivation.
Just shows up and gets it done.
That's not discipline.
That's identity.

Stack the Day, Not the Dream.

Forget the five-year plan.
Forget the fantasy version of your future self.
You only ever live one day at a time - so build that one well.
Stop chasing visions if you keep tripping over your mornings.
Look at today.
Not, "*Someday.*"

Did you earn your pillow tonight?
Did you move forward or drift?
The dream is just fiction if today's a mess.
But if you win today, and win it again tomorrow?
That's how real momentum starts.
Self-respect, confidence and clarity all follow one thing...
Consistency.

Audit the Autopilot.

Most of your life happens without conscious choice.
Which means your defaults better be lock, stock, and loaded.
So audit them.
Ruthlessly.
What's the first thing you reach for when you're tired?
What do you do when no one's telling you what to do?
Where do your thoughts go when your focus slips?
How do you respond when no one's pushing you?
These aren't throwaway moments.
They're the scaffolding of your entire existence.
And if your autopilot is built on junk, comfort, distraction, and cheap dopamine hits, don't be shocked when you keep circling the same dead ends.
Rewire that shit.
Because you'll never out-affirm a broken loop.

The Environment Multiplier.

Habits don't exist in isolation.
They live inside an ecosystem - one that's either feeding your growth or strangling it.
You could have the sharpest morning routine, the clearest goals, the strongest intentions…
But if your environment is working against you?
Good luck!
You're trying to eat clean while your fridge is full of Creme Eggs.
Trying to focus while your phone claws at your attention.
Trying to level up while the people around you treat ambition like a punchline.
Sure, discipline matters - but environment is the multiplier.

If your space is messy, your thoughts will be too.
If your phone is a portal to bullshit, your focus doesn't stand a chance.
If your circle mocks effort, you'll shrink to belong.
You don't rise above your surroundings, you adapt to them.
You can't game psychology.
So set your space up like your future depends on it.
Put your phone in another room when you need deep focus.
Organise your kitchen for health, not temptation.
Curate your digital inputs like your mental bandwidth is currency.
Spend time with people who stretch you - not the ones who soothe your mediocrity.
You don't just need better habits.
You need a habitat that supports them.
One that reflects who you're becoming - not who you're trying to outgrow.

The Loop That Builds (or Breaks) You.

Every time you follow through on a promise to yourself - even a small one - you make a deposit into your self-respect.
That's the loop that builds you.
You act.

You reinforce trust.
You act again.
And eventually?
Confidence becomes default.
Self-belief becomes muscle memory.
No permission required.
But every time you flake?
Every time you bail on your own word?
You train your brain to expect disappointment.
Not from the world - from you.
That's the loop most people quietly die in.
Not from laziness.
Not from lack of effort.
But from the slow erosion of belief.
It starts small -
"I'll start tomorrow."
"I'll just skip today."
"I'm too tired."
And before you realise it, the identity you wanted has been replaced by one that doubts itself.
You don't need another reset.
You don't need another hype cycle.
You need receipts.
Reps.
Proof.
You need to stack the wins until your nervous system no longer questions your commitment.
And become someone whose word is law, even when no one's watching.
Because when you stop needing outside validation to feel proud of how you move?
That's when you're dangerous.
That's when you're free.

Put It On the Table.

Does this 'thought' hit home?
☐ Yes   ☐ Not really

If yes, can you call yourself out and apply it?
☐ Yes   ☐ Still hiding

If yes, what's one move you'll make to prove it's not just words?

....

....

Thought 17
Put Your White Belt Back On.

You did it.
You got good at something.
You climbed the mountain.
You earned your stripes.
Maybe even got a few people calling you an expert.

Congrats.

Now take that black belt off.
Fold it neatly.
And put the white one back on.
Because real killers don't sit at the top polishing trophies.
They don't camp at the summit, clinging to past peaks.
They find the next mountain.
And start climbing again - with bleeding hands and zero ego.

Success Is a Trap if You Let It Be.

The most dangerous words in growth?
"Completed it mate."
"That's beneath me."
"I don't need to learn that."
Those aren't the thoughts of a champion.
They're the thoughts of someone who's plateaued but too proud to admit it.
You know who else thought they were untouchable?

Nokia.
Blockbuster.
Skype.
And that one mate who peaked in uni, still quoting freshers' week 'bants', now spending his weekends signing on, getting stoned, and retelling the same three stories about when he was 'the man.'
You think you're built for more?
Then prove it.
Not by staying on top - but by starting again.
By being shit at something new.
By letting go of the applause and choosing growth instead.

The Cost of Competence.

Getting good at something feels incredible - until it becomes your prison.
When people start clapping, you stop experimenting.
When you start getting paid for it, you stop playing with it.
What used to be fun becomes a reputation to protect.
You stop swinging for the fences.
You start protecting what you already have.
You shift from creation to maintenance.
That's the cost of competence.
You get so wrapped up in being known for something, you forget how to grow at anything.

That's how talent turns stale.
That's how sharp people get soft.
They confuse mastery with arrival.
But real mastery?
It's built by those who keep asking -
"What else don't I know yet?"
"Where am I rusty?"
"Where am I coasting?"
The moment you fear looking like a beginner again...
That's the moment your decline begins.

Humility Isn't Weakness, It's Fuel.

Walking into a room where you're the worst one there?
That's not shameful.
That's sacred.
It means you've got something to learn.
It means you've stepped out of the shallow end.
It means you're exactly where you're supposed to be.
Real growth starts the moment you're willing to suck again.
When you're willing to feel uncomfortable.
When your confidence takes a hit, but your curiosity stays standing.
When you trade ego for exposure, because you know the long game isn't status.
It's strength.
The people who last?
They chase humility like oxygen.
Because they know that the moment you're *"too good"* to start over...
You're done.

Comfort Is the Slowest Death Imaginable.

You mastered your craft?
Cool.
Now switch lanes.
You're strong in the gym?
Learn to dance.
You crushed it in business?
Try painting.
You've got speaking gigs?
Take a silent retreat.
If you're always the sharpest one in the room, you're in the wrong room.
Comfort is a sedative.
It whispers, "Stay here. You've made it."
Then it buries you in sameness and slow decline.

You've got to feel like a fraud again.

You've got to sweat before trying something new.
Get shaky.
Get humbled.
Fall flat.
Laugh louder.
That's how you stay dangerous.
Because when you're willing to eat dirt again, no one can hold you hostage with comfort.

You Flex, You're Fucked.

There's a term in martial arts - 'Shoshin'.
Beginner's mind.
It's about approaching everything, even what you already know, through the eyes of a rookie.
Because the second you think you've *"arrived"* - you've stopped moving.
So keep white belt energy.
Ask dumb questions.
Take criticism on the chin.
Stay curious, not cocky.
Stay raw, not rehearsed.
Keep learning, even when it's ugly.

White belt energy doesn't mean weak.
It means you're still hunting.
Still nimble.
Still dangerous.
It means you're not just growing - you're building to outlast.

I'm Sat Here Writing a Book.

It's 9:53 p.m.
My daughter's asleep (for now).
And I'm sat on my couch in Manchester writing a book.
A fucking book.

I cheated my way to a C in GCSE English, and now I'm banging out 'thoughts' like I belong here in my aggressive Mancunian tone of voice.
I send them to my old dear to check over...
She hates it.
Thinks the swearing's too much, and the tone too harsh.
But I'm doing it anyway.
Not because I think I'm a good writer.
Because I'm a shit one and I'm writing anyway.

That's white belt energy.
That's what this 'thought' is all about.
Doing the thing before you're good at it.
Leaning in when your inner critic says, *"Who the fuck do you think you are?"*
That voice never goes away.
You just stop letting it drive.

Your Comfort Zone Will Murder Your Potential.

Most people get good enough - then park.
They coast on praise.
Rewatch their highlight reel.
And die a slow death of mediocrity with a smirk on their face and potential still in the tank.
But not you.
Put your white belt back on.
Be shit at something.
Feel the sting of not knowing.
Ask for help.
Miss the shot.
Own the mistake.
Keep swinging anyway.

That's how you become a savage in the long term.
Not by proving you're already great.

But by chasing what might make you greater.
That's not weakness.
That's legacy thinking.

Put It On the Table.

Does this 'thought' hit home?
☐ Yes　☐ Not really

If yes, can you call yourself out and apply it?
☐ Yes　☐ Still hiding

If yes, what's one move you'll make to prove it's not just words?

....

....

Thought 18
You Owe Your Future Self a Fight.

There's a version of you out there.
Older, uglier, slightly better at folding fitted sheets.
You'll meet them one day - give them something to thank you for.
Because whether that future version is built or broken depends on what you do right now.
Every moment you delay, scroll, settle, or self-sabotage - that version of you pays the price.
This isn't abstract.
It's not theory.
It's real.
And that future you is watching.
Waiting.
Silently asking one question - *"Are you going to fight for me? Or fold?"*

Every Choice Is a Vote for the Person You'll Become.

You think skipping the workout is no big deal?
You think putting off that side hustle is just a pause?
You think that skinny line of Charlie is harmless fun?
You're wrong.
It's all cumulative.
Because every micro-decision is either a seed or a thief.
Every choice feeds your future or robs it.
You're either paying into your potential or borrowing against it.
Discipline today means freedom tomorrow.

Avoidance today means regret tomorrow.
It's a brutal exchange rate - and there's no refund counter.
Greatness isn't made in single grand gestures.
It's built from the moments nobody sees.
When it's late and you're tired.
When no one's checking in.
When quitting would be easier and entirely justifiable.
That's where futures are forged.

People Plan for Retirement - Why Not Their Character?

We spend more time thinking about pensions than we do purpose.
We prepare to be solvent in our sixties but rarely ask whether we'll be proud of who we've become.
You'll meet your future self with more than a bank balance.
You'll bring them your habits.
Your regrets.
Your track record.
Your integrity.
Will they thank you?
Or sit across from you with quiet resentment?
That's the real retirement question.
That's the real fight.
And no, you can't outsource this.
You can't invest your way into courage.
You can't borrow grit from a coach or an influencer.
No one is coming to gift you a backbone.
You build it. Or you don't.
And one day, you'll have to live with the result…
In the mirror.
In your mind.
In the moment you realise who you became… was entirely up to you.

The Version of You That's Worth Meeting.

You want to meet the version of you who keeps promises to

themselves.
Shows up when it's not sexy.
Gets back up after taking hits.
Builds things instead of just dreaming about them.
Carries quiet pride, even when no one's watching.
That version of you doesn't show up by accident.
They're not born out of vibes, motivation, or good intentions.
They only exist if you fight for them now.
Not tomorrow.
Now.
You don't drift into greatness.
You don't stumble into peace.
You don't accidentally become someone you respect.
You fight your way there.

What You Avoid Today, They Inherit Tomorrow.

The hard conversations you dodge?
They'll deal with the fallout.
The health you neglect?
They carry the cost.
The work you skip?
They get stuck cleaning it up.
The dreams you bury?
They live with the "*what ifs.*"
That future version of you doesn't need your excuses.
They don't need your rationale.
They need your discipline.
Your focus.
Your uncompromising refusal to coast.

The Quiet Currency of Effort.

There's no app that tracks it.
No notification when you've made a deposit.
But every time you do the thing you'd rather avoid, you're putting

credit in a future account.
And one day - when life tries to bankrupt you - that account will matter.
That's the quiet currency of effort.
It won't trend.
It won't shine.
But it will hold you together.
When the storms hit.
When the lights go out.
When nobody's watching and everything feels pointless.
You'll be standing.
Not because you had better luck, more time, or natural talent -
But because you paid in advance.

Make Them Proud to Carry Your Name.

Future you isn't a concept.
They're real.
With your name.
Your memories.
Your scars.
Your reputation.
One day, they'll sit across from someone and be asked -
"What made you who you are?"
Make sure they don't answer with -
"I gave up."
"I waited until I felt ready."
"I wasted years avoiding the work."
Give them stories worth telling.
Habits worth passing on.
A spine built from your current effort.
Because whether you see it or not, everything you do right now echoes.

Leave Them Something Worth Carrying.

The fight you take on today might be invisible.
No audience. No applause. No payoff in sight.
That's fine.
Because your future self will know.
They'll feel it in their backbone.
In the moments when things get heavy - and they don't break.
That strength comes from you.
Right now.
Right here.
Don't leave them your debts.
Your chaos.
Your avoidance.
Your half-finished promises.
Leave them your legacy.
Give them something to stand on, not something to dig out of.
You owe them that.
So start paying up.

Put It On the Table.

Does this 'thought' hit home?
☐ Yes   ☐ Not really

If yes, can you call yourself out and apply it?
☐ Yes   ☐ Still hiding

If yes, what's one move you'll make to prove it's not just words?

....

....

Part 3

BURN THE OLD SCRIPT

Thought 19
Your Circle Is Your Ceiling.

Let's not fuck about, this one's going to cut deep.
Your circle will either build you or break you.
Let that land.
Not your education.
Not your background.
Not your bank account.
Not even your talent.
It's who you keep closest.

They shape more than your schedule.
They shape your standards.
Your beliefs.
Your sense of what's possible.
So if you're feeling stuck, heavy, or like you're grinding but never getting lift…
Maybe it's not your strategy.
Maybe it's your people.

Look Around Before You Look Ahead.

Everyone's chasing their next level.
Grinding.
Manifesting.
Building their 'best self'.
But here's what most won't say out loud -
You can't rise surrounded by anchors.
Try sprinting with a backpack full of bricks.

That's what it feels like evolving next to people who stay static.
Who flinch at change.
Who pretend to support you, but only until your wins start making them uncomfortable.
They'll say they've got your back, but it's just to make sure you don't get too far ahead.
They'll smile when you win, but it won't touch their eyes.
They'll joke about your goals, then shrug and say "*Just messing.*"
But you'll feel it.
That energy.
That edge.
Because your growth pokes their fear.
And instead of facing it, they try to drag you back to the old rhythm.
The one that kept them safe.
The one you outgrew.

Loyalty Isn't Shrinking for Someone Else's Comfort.

We're taught early to stick by our people.
"*No new friends.*"
"*Don't forget where you came from.*"
"*Ride or die.*"
It sounds noble.
Feels loyal.
But if sticking with your day ones means suffocating your next chapter, that's not loyalty.
That's slow-motion sabotage.

Some people were meant for a moment.
A season.
A version of you that no longer fits.
And that's okay.
You don't have to vilify someone to realise you've outgrown them.
Growth is supposed to change your circle.
That's not a betrayal of your past.
It's a commitment to your future.

Familiar Doesn't Mean Safe.

The people slowing you down rarely look like a threat.
Sometimes, they just look like home.
Comfortable.
Familiar.
The friend who's always down for a drink, but never down for a deep conversation.
The cousin who tells the same three stories every time you mention trying something new.
The colleague who complains about fucking everything but never changes anything.
They're not bad people.
But they're not building anything either.
And that matters.
Because if you stay too long in that environment, you won't even realise you've built a padded cell.
Lined with nostalgia, low standards, and good intentions.
It won't feel dangerous.
It'll feel warm.
That's how slow decline works - it feels safe while it starves you.
You'll start lowering your goals just to fit in.
You'll silence your ideas to avoid making them uncomfortable.
And one day, you'll wake up more liked than respected.
That's when the guilt kicks in.
Because these are people you care about.
It's tempting to stay, to shrink, just to keep the peace.
You don't have to hate them.
But you do have to face the truth -
They're not pushing you forward.
They're just making you feel okay with standing still.

You Can't Win Surrounded by Losers.

I'm not talking about money, status, or Instagram followers.
I'm talking about mindset.

If your circle rolls their eyes when you talk about growth?
If they treat your ambition like a punchline or a threat?
If every win you share gets met with sarcasm instead of celebration?
You're not in a circle.
You're in a cage.
Winners don't belittle people chasing better.
They study it.
They share strategies.
They clap loudly.
They say, "*Fuck yeah, how can I help?*"
Losers?
They minimise.
Mock.
Sabotage.
And they'll hide behind "*just a laugh*" while they're clipping your wings.
Because your progress shines a light on what they're avoiding.
And instead of levelling up, they'd rather pull you down.
If someone needs you to stay small for them to feel okay?
That's not friendship.
That's ego management.

Build a Table You'd Bleed With.

Here's the only metric that matters -
Can you win big and not feel like you have to shrink?
Can you fail and not feel judged?
Can you cry and still be seen as strong?
If not - you're not at the right table.
Your people should remind you who the fuck you are when you forget.
They challenge you when you play small.
They sit with your pain without trying to fix it.

And when you're crawling, doubting, falling apart - they don't stand
over you with advice.
They don't offer clichés or platitudes.
They get on the floor, lock eyes, and say -
"*We're not fucking done yet.*"

That's your circle.

Outgrowing Isn't Abandonment.

Some of the people you love the most will not come with you.
They'll mock your change.
Punish your clarity.
Cling to the version of you that made them feel okay.
And when you keep growing, they'll call it betrayal.
They'll say - *"You've changed."*
Damn right.
That's the whole point.

But listen - you're not abandoning them.
You're refusing to abandon yourself.
History is not a good enough reason to stay stuck.
Just because someone was there when you were broke, broken, or bouncing between bad decisions doesn't mean they've earned a lifetime seat at your table.
Not everyone grows at the same pace.
Not everyone wants to.
You don't build your future by dragging the past behind you like a trophy.
You build it by being honest about what no longer fits, and having the guts to let it go.

Guilt Is Not a Sign to Stay.

Here's why good people get stuck - guilt.
We confuse wanting more with being disloyal.
We shrink ourselves to keep the peace.
We carry others' comfort on our backs and call it loyalty.
But that's not loyalty.
That's emotional hostage-taking - and you're the one in cuffs.
Real loyalty respects growth.

It doesn't resist when your standards rise.
It doesn't guilt you for evolving.
It grows with you, or cheers you on from afar.
True loyalty doesn't demand proximity.
It demands truth.
The real ones don't panic when you change.
They pivot. They adjust. They ask how they can support.
And if they can't?
They bow out with love.
But the wrong ones?
They'll try to shame you back into your old self.
They'll call your boundaries selfish.
Your clarity arrogance.
Your peace a problem.

You don't owe anyone a diluted version of yourself.
You owe yourself a life that feels like truth.
A rhythm that fits who you are now - not who they liked better.
And if someone can't handle who you're becoming?
That's on them.
Your job is to keep going - even if it rattles the ones still standing still.
Let them talk.
Let them misunderstand you.
Let them miss the old you.
Your results will do the answering.

Be Your Own Circle Until the Right One Finds You.

If you've cut loose the old crew and haven't found your new one yet -
that's okay.
This in-between is sacred.
Be your own mirror.
Be your own hype team.
Be your own standard-setter.
This part might feel lonely, but it's not empty - it's foundational.
You're setting the tone for the energy you'll allow in.
You're building a version of you that doesn't beg for belonging.

The right people will show up -
Not when you're desperate, but when you're whole.
Until then, don't dim your fire just to feel less alone.
Burn so bright they find you by the light.

Put It On the Table.

Does this 'thought' hit home?
☐ Yes ☐ Not really

If yes, can you call yourself out and apply it?
☐ Yes ☐ Still hiding

If yes, what's one move you'll make to prove it's not just words?

....

....

Thought 20
Kings Without Kingdoms.

Everyone wants to be a king these days.
It's in the bios.
It's in the reels.
It's barked across podcasts like gospel.
Here's where most people get it twisted -
Crowns don't come from clout.
And no, your bank account, your six-pack, or your follower count
don't qualify.
A real kingdom isn't measured in attention.
It's measured in impact.
It's not how many people know your name, it's how many people are
better because you showed up.
You don't build a kingdom through self-promotion.
You build it by holding weight no one else will touch.
And doing it without needing thanks.

Kings Don't Flex - They Carry Weight.

We've glamorised the image of influencer royalty.
Gold watches.
Private jets.
Women orbiting like accessories.
But that isn't kingship.
It's male fragility in Gucci mink yelling about being *"high value"*.
A true king doesn't lead with aesthetics.
He leads with actions.
He doesn't walk in the room needing to be loud.
He brings clarity with his silence.

His presence brings calm.
His decisions bring direction.
He carries what others drop.
He absorbs pressure, protects the vulnerable, and shows up consistently - especially when it's inconvenient.

Being a king isn't about looking important, it's about being responsible.
You can call yourself royalty all day long.
But if nobody feels safer, stronger, or more stable in your presence, you're not leading.
You're pretending.
Because if you're not lifting others, you're just a boy in a borrowed crown.

The Crown Isn't Shiny, It's Heavy.

A crown isn't a trophy.
It's a weight.
It doesn't sit gently.
It presses into your skin.
It means showing up when you're exhausted.
It means choosing discipline when your emotions scream otherwise.
It means staying grounded while everything around you spins.

Real kings bleed behind the scenes.
They sacrifice privately.
They carry storms so others don't drown in them.
They make decisions that cost them peace - because protecting others matters more than their own comfort.
And when nobody's watching?
They don't slip.
They don't fold.
They still hold the line.
Leadership isn't loud.
It's not about barking orders.
It's about who you are when there's no applause, no reward, no

recognition.
Anyone can lead when it's easy.
Kings lead when it's hard.
So if your version of manhood is domination without duty, power without principle, swagger without sacrifice -
Then you're not a king.
You're just hiding behind bravado.

What Are You Actually Building?

What do you actually lead?
What have you created that serves anyone beyond your own ego?
Because being a king means -
Legacy.
Stability.
Future-proof structures.
Not just financial security, but moral scaffolding.
Emotional safety.
A place where others stop bracing for impact because your steadiness rewrote the atmosphere.
If all you've built is a brand...
If your kingdom is just a curated identity, stitched together from borrowed quotes and your best lighting...
Then you've missed the assignment.

True kings plant trees they'll never sit under.
They build castles not just for their own comfort, but for others' protection.
They create space for growth, for family, for friends, for community.
No legacy was ever built off self-promotion alone.
Your last post might get a load of engagement, but your actual life?
That's the only thing people will remember.

Start With the Castle Walls.

Don't talk about being a king if your own house is a disaster.

If your habits are erratic.
If your promises mean nothing.
If the people closest to you are walking on eggshells.
You want to lead?
Start with the foundation.
Start at home.
Make your home a place of peace, not tension.
Make your word a source of trust, not suspicion.
Make your habits so reliable they become a shelter for others.

Before you try to rule anything, learn how to rule yourself.
That means confronting your compulsions.
That means pausing before you unload.
That means choosing silence when rage would be easier.
Because kings don't chase every urge.
They don't let their shadow run the show.
They know when to speak, and when to shut the fuck up.
That kind of inner governance?
It's not glamorous.
But it's rare.
And it's powerful.
Because people will only follow a man who has mastered himself.

Kings Don't Outsource Their Battles.

Being a leader means fighting battles others never see.
You don't get to blame your past for every reaction.
You don't get to outsource your triggers to the people you love.
Being a king means owning your story.
It means facing your wounds without handing out blame.
It means holding your anger, your fear, your mess, and doing
something useful with it.
It's not about being flawless.
It's about being accountable.
Because if your loved ones are paying the price for your unhealed shit,
you're not leading - you're leaking.

A real king does the internal work.
He turns his pain into clarity.
He walks into the emotional fire so his circle doesn't have to.
And he doesn't broadcast it for credit.
He just does it.

Kings Don't Starve Their People.

You can't call yourself a king if the people around you are starving.
Not just for money - for presence.
Encouragement.
Wisdom.
Patience.
If your leadership sucks the life out of people instead of lighting something within them, you're not just falling short - you're feeding off the very people you're meant to fortify.
Real kings pour into others.
They teach.
They empower.
They call out greatness and then show you how to live it.
They know that feeding others doesn't diminish their strength, it multiplies it.
A true king doesn't build a spotlight.
He builds a shelter.
A place where others breathe easier, grow faster, and stop bracing for chaos.
Because true leadership isn't how much you collect - it's how much you contribute.
And if your kingdom is built entirely around your needs, then it's not a kingdom.
It's a cult of one.

Crowns Are Earned, Not Claimed.

You don't become a king because someone gives you a title.

You become a king the moment you start living like one - long before anyone notices.
Character over comfort.
Service over status.
Legacy over lust.
You earn it when you put principles before preferences.
When you stop chasing image and start embodying purpose.

So next time you see someone stomping through social media, barking about how alpha they are - ask one question -
Where's your kingdom, bro?
Not the props.
Not the car.
The kingdom.
Where are the people thriving because of your leadership?
Where's the family, the team, that's been elevated by your presence?
If they can't answer that?
They're not a king.
They're just a fucking sausage playing dress-up in their reality of 'red pill' fuckery.

Put It On the Table.

Does this 'thought' hit home?
☐ Yes   ☐ Not really

If yes, can you call yourself out and apply it?
☐ Yes   ☐ Still hiding

If yes, what's one move you'll make to prove it's not just words?

....

....

Thought 21
If It's Not a Hell Yeah, It's a Fuck Off.

Most of your stress doesn't come from overwork.
It comes from betrayal.
Not from others, but by yourself.
Every time you override your instincts, you abandon yourself a little more.
It starts subtly.
You accept the job that didn't sit right.
Say yes to the catch-up you weren't excited about.
Join the project that felt off from the beginning.
Agree to the invite out of politeness.
You show up, play along, nod and smile - all while your gut's waving red flags like it's trying to save your life.
But you override it.
You rationalise.
You compromise.
You tell yourself it'll be fine.
And it's not.
Because every time you say yes to something you don't really want, you're not just being nice - you're shrinking your soul.

The Slow Death of Maybe.

You don't lose your life in some sort of dramatic nosedive.
It erodes.
Quietly.
Death by a thousand polite nods.

You say "yes" when your whole body whispers "no".
You don't feel the fracture at first.
But you're not at ease - and it shows in your energy.
Over time, your life turns beige.
A job that kind of sucks, but not enough to quit.
A relationship that feels like wallpaper.
A calendar full of events you secretly hope get cancelled.
You scroll through it all in a trance - half present, half resentful.
From the outside, it looks fine.
No disaster.
No crisis.
Just muted.
A sad little mime.

Comfort becomes complacency.
"It could be worse" becomes your baseline.
That's mediocrity.
And it doesn't scream.
It whispers.
"Settle.
It's safer."
But it's not safe.
It's slow suffocation.

Your Gut Already Knows.

Your body always knows before your brain catches up.
That tight chest when the invite comes in?
That's not anxiety.
That's clarity.
That urge to scroll, escape, distract?
That's a signal.
That quiet little "eugh" when a name pops up on your phone?
That's truth.
But we override it.
We're taught to be nice.
To be grateful.

To be agreeable.
We swallow our instincts to avoid disappointing others.
Meanwhile, we disappoint ourselves.
Again and again.
We teach ourselves that "*no*" is mean.
That honesty is rude.
That gut feelings are irrational.
So we smiled we nod like a dog and keep saying "*yes*".
And with every one, we shrink.
Here's the rule, plain and simple...
If it's not a full body "*yes*", it's a "*fuck off*".
You don't need logic.
You don't need to justify it.
You don't need a reason to honour your own clarity.

No Is a Superpower.

Saying "*no*" isn't rejection.
It's reclamation.
Every "*no*" gives you back time.
Back energy.
Back space.
Every "*no*" draws a boundary in bold -
"*This is who I am. This is what I want. This is what I won't tolerate.*"
It's not cruelty.
It's clarity.
And yeah, honesty can sting.
But it stings clean.
It clears the air instead of clouding it.
It cuts through the static.
You don't need to soften it with twenty disclaimers.
Try this -
"*Thanks for thinking of me, but I'm focusing elsewhere.*"
"*Appreciate it, but I'm going to pass.*"
"*No.*"
That last one?
That's a full sentence.

Use it.

Build a Life You Don't Want to Escape.

Most people plan their holidays like it's the only relief they get from their life.
That's a red flag.
If you're fantasising about escape more than you're excited about your day?
Red flag.
Imagine waking up and thinking *"Hell yeah."*
Not to everything.
But to enough.
To work that challenges you, not bleeds you dry.
To people who stretch you, not shrink you.
To projects that feel like play, not performance.
To stillness that fills you, not boredom you have to numb with content.
This isn't about perfection. It's about presence.
That full-blooded, clear-eyed presence that says, *"This life? I chose it."*

You don't need a yacht or a breakthrough.
You just need to stop tolerating what quietly kills your spirit.
Joy doesn't come from accumulation. It comes from alignment.
That's the real work.
Not adding more to your life, but stripping away what was never yours to begin with.

Hell Yeah or Noise.

A *"Hell yeah"* takes guts.
Because it means you're all in.
And you can't be all in if half your heart is stuck in things you don't even like.
You want clarity?
Cut the background noise.
You want power?

Stop bleeding it out on people and projects you've already outgrown. You'll be shocked at how fast life sharpens when you stop managing other people's comfort and start honouring your own truth.

Between Hell Yeah and Fuck Off Lives the Real You.

Not everyone will love this version of you.
Some people will flinch.
Some will ghost.
Some will talk shit.

Fuck 'em.

Some people are only there to keep you average.
If your clarity scares them, that's their invitation to exit.
The ones who respect it?
They'll ride with you.
This is your life.
Your stage.
Your headliner set.
Don't waste it on *"meh."*
Don't say *"yes"* just because you're afraid to say *"no"*.
If it doesn't make your blood sing, it's not yours.
Let it go.

Put It On the Table.

Does this 'thought' hit home?
☐ Yes   ☐ Not really

If yes, can you call yourself out and apply it?
☐ Yes   ☐ Still hiding

If yes, what's one move you'll make to prove it's not just words?

....

....

Thought 22
Not Everything Deserves a Reaction.

You don't need to bark when you know you've got teeth.
We live in a culture wired to clap back.
Say something slick, throw a jab online, drop a passive-aggressive
dig. And the masses scramble to quote, post, explain.
Everyone wants the last word.
Everyone wants to be seen swinging.
But every reaction is a leak.
A drain.
A loss.

You think you're standing up for yourself, but really you're spending
yourself.
Every time you respond to nonsense, you're cutting a slice of your
energy and handing it out to people who haven't earned it.
Most of the world's running on emotional overdraft.
Burning out over bullshit that shouldn't even be on their radar.
They want your attention, they want your reaction.
Because a reaction tells them you're controllable.

You give up control every time you react.
You prove you're reachable.
Pullable.
Playable.
And the second people see that?
Game on.
The ones who really move the needle?
They don't react.

They don't perform.
They don't justify.
They go quiet.
They tighten their shoes.
They know silence isn't surrender - it's a loaded gun with the safety off.

Reactivity Exposes You.

In poker, a 'tell' gives away your off suit seven-deuce.
Same in life.
Every time you take the bait, you're handing them your blueprint.
You're saying, *"Here's how to pull my strings."*
Some people will use that to manipulate you.
Others just like the chaos.
Others don't even know why they're poking the bear - they just like the noise.
Once they know where to press, they'll press.
Again and again.
Reactivity isn't resistance - it's broadcast.
You're showing them how to play you.
Real power isn't in a killer comeback.
It's in not needing to show up for the fight at all.

Impulse Isn't Strength. It's Weakness in Motion.

Anyone can fire off a tweet.
Anyone can send a heated text, record a rant, hit send on a story.
That's not courage - that's compulsion.
The real work is in the pause.
That brutal second where your ego flares and you don't let it drive.
Where you feel the sting and you don't bleed out over it.

Instead, you breathe.
You ask - Is this noise, or something real?
Maturity is in that breath.

It's in swallowing the urge and sitting with the heat.
Not to deny it but to decide if it's worth bleeding for.
Nine times out of ten, it's not.

Your Focus Is Gold.

Not every insult needs a reply.
Not every shade thrown deserves a spotlight.
Not every person gets a seat at your emotional table.
Your attention is currency and if you're handing it out like free
samples, don't be surprised when your peace feels broke.
Reacting to everything feels like power.
It's not.
It's a nervous tic dressed up as purpose.
Big alpha vibes… bless its fragile heart.
Be selective.
Be selfish with your energy.
You've got better things to build.

Silence Is Not Absence.

Silence isn't checking out.
It's zoning in.
It's not 'being the bigger person.'
It's being the smarter one.
It's pulling back from battles that don't move your life forward - from
dramas that eat time and leave nothing in their wake.
Think of reactions as strings.
Every time you bite, someone's playing you like a budget Punch and
Judy.
Silence?
That's you shutting the curtain, burning the stage, and sending the
puppets home in a Tesco bag.

You're not avoiding.
You're hunting bigger game.

You're tuned so far into your mission that petty doesn't even register on your radar.
Let them misread you.
Let them invent stories.
You've got better things to build than your reputation in the mouths of small thinkers.

Your Peace Isn't Public Property.

Some people demand reactions like it's owed to them.
As if your silence is an insult.
Let them squirm.
Let them throw tantrums in your absence.
Let them think they've won because you didn't show up.
You don't owe anyone your centre just because they're spinning out.
Chaos will always try to seduce your attention.
You stay cold.
You stay focused.
You stay building.

While they're talking, you're stacking.
While they're watching, you're working.
While they're pushing buttons, you're unplugging the whole system.

Let Them Choke on the Silence.

You don't owe explanations.
You don't owe reactions.
You don't have to correct every misread or defend every move.
Let them wonder.
Let them talk themselves in circles trying to figure out why you didn't bite.
You're not here to be understood.
You're here to live clean.
Sharp.
Unapologetic.

You're not chasing arguments.
You're chasing legacy.

Training the Pause.

The pause won't come easy or naturally at first.
You've spent years reacting on instinct.
Flinch.
Snap.
Defend.
That's how we are programmed to survive.

Now you train new reflexes.
Count to three.
Breathe through the heat.
Let the first thought die before it reaches your mouth.
Run the play even when your blood's boiling.
Step back.
Go walk.
Write the angry text and don't send it.
Turn the phone off.

Don't feed the beast.
The voice that says "*do something*"?
Ignore it.
Starve it into silence.
The one that says "*let it go*"?
That's the one you strengthen.
Every time you choose silence, you're not bottling it - you're building it.
And in that silence, you become lethal.
Controlled.
Cold-blooded calm.
Not because you're weak.
Because you're fucking dangerous when you're focused.

Speak Only When It Hits Like a Bat.

You don't need to clap back to hold your ground.
You don't need to match mess with mess.
You don't need to say a fucking word.
Let them talk.
Let them flail.
Let them exhaust themselves in the noise.
Because silence is a power move.
Not passive - precise.
Not timid - tactical.
You don't lose power by staying quiet - you conserve it.
And when you do speak?
Make it count.
Make it land like Lucille.

Put It On the Table.

Does this 'thought' hit home?
☐ Yes   ☐ Not really

If yes, can you call yourself out and apply it?
☐ Yes   ☐ Still hiding

If yes, what's one move you'll make to prove it's not just words?

....

....

Thought 23
Choose the Target, Ignore the Crowd.

Once you've locked in, nothing else matters.
Not the claps.
Not the glances.
Not the opinions.

Look straight.
Breathe.

The moment you start scanning the room, you lose speed.
Most people don't stall because they're soft - they stall because they're addicted to being noticed.
They need reaction.
Feedback.
A nod from the gallery.
Like their goals aren't real unless someone claps.
But attention isn't fuel - it's friction.
And the crowd doesn't kill your momentum.
Your need to be seen does.

Opinions Are Like Arseholes.

The second you commit to something real, out come the experts fresh off doing fuck all.
Suddenly the guy juggling Klarna payments is dishing out investment advice.
The one who's never built a thing in their life wants to workshop your

business plan.

And the bloke who ghosted his own goals is full of *"just being honest"* takes about your discipline.

They're not critiquing you - they're comforting themselves.

Because every step you take forward reminds them they're standing still.

The louder your actions, the louder their commentary.

That's not coincidence - it's physics mate. And I got a U at A-Level.

Movement = friction.

If they're not carrying your weight, they don't get a say in how you move.

If they're not building what you're building, they're just spectators.

And spectators don't shape outcomes, they heckle from the stands.

Stop Explaining.

Your evolution doesn't need permission.

Your ambition doesn't need a fucking monologue.

You're not an exhibit.

You're not a committee decision.

The second you stop performing your old self, people panic.

Not because you're wrong, but because you prove change is a choice.

And that's threatening to those who never made one.

You say *"no"* when you used to say *"yes"*.

You train while they drink.

You invest while they coast.

You shed the version they were comfortable with and they call it arrogance.

They say you've changed.

They say you're intense.

They say you think you're better.

You're not trying to be better than them.

You're just not interested in being like them.

You Don't Need Validation. You Need Focus.

You don't need to post it for it to be real.
You don't need every move witnessed, liked, or shared.
You're not an influencer - you're building for impact.
And that often means disappearing.
Going deeper.
Going dark while your work gets louder.

Let them misread your silence.
Let them confuse your absence for arrogance.
Because when the dust settles?
They'll be sitting in the same place - and you'll have built something they can't ignore.
The ones who get it?
They're too deep in their own grind to give a fuck about your relatability.
You're not here to be understood.
You're here to be undeniable.

Respect Doesn't Always Come With Familiarity.

As you rise, being understood becomes rare.
You'll speak less.
Exit more rooms.
Cut ties with noise.
And it will land like a wet fart.
Because your clarity exposes their drift.
Your discipline shines a light on their delay.

They won't admit it, but you'll feel it.
The snide comments.
The shade wrapped in 'balance' advice.
All attempts to pull you back to where they felt equal.
Don't bite.
Don't shrink.

You're not here to be digestible.
Let them wrestle with the version of you they no longer control.

You Can't Build Legacy in a Popularity Contest.

You'll never build something lasting if you're addicted to being liked.
Legacy doesn't care about followers - it cares about footprint.
And that comes at a cost most won't pay.
Building something real - your business, your body, your boundaries -
means stepping out of the spotlight and into the furnace.
No filters.
No validation.
Just you and the uncomfortable truth.

Growth is gritty.
It's quiet.
It's endless repetition.
It's hard choices made in silence.
It's progress that no one cares about until it's done.
Meanwhile, the world's throwing parties for mediocrity.
And if you're not careful, you'll start mistaking popularity for progress.
But the work that makes you legendary?
It doesn't trend.
It goes deep.
It compounds in the dark.
You don't get remembered for playing to the crowd.
You get remembered for building something that outlives their
attention span.

Loud Isn't the Same as Legendary.

Everyone's yelling.
Everyone's selling.
Everyone's got a brand, a bio, a fucking slogan.
They're curating themselves into content.
Polishing their bollocks for an audience that forgets by lunchtime.

But volume doesn't equal value.
Being loud doesn't make you legendary - it just makes you obvious.
And obvious fades fast.

Real greatness moves differently.
It's not crafted in Canva or cut for reels.
It's forged in pressure.
It's carved through standards.
Legend isn't built in the moment - it's built across many.
Through consistency, through pressure and through outcomes that speak louder than your marketing ever could.
Because legacy doesn't need to trend.
It doesn't give a fuck about how many tuned in - only who walked away changed.
That's the difference.
Influence tries to be seen.
Impact ensures it's felt.
Let them master the algorithm.
You master your craft.
Let them build audiences.
You build foundations.

Make the Move - Whether They See It or Not.

Not every step needs an audience.
Not every decision needs defending.
You're not seeking permission.
You're applying pressure.
So move like no one's watching and like your results will be impossible to ignore.

Let them assume you're proving a point.
You're not.
You're just aligning your life with your potential, and that makes the crowd twitch.

Approval Will Water Down Your Fire.

Every time you hesitate to keep people comfortable, you lose sharpness.
Every time you ask, *"Will they get it?"* you dilute your edge.
Before long, you're reshaping bold instincts into safe moves.
You're rounding corners that were never meant to be soft.
Execution doesn't need validation.
It needs clarity.
It needs conviction.
The approval you're chasing is coming from people who couldn't handle your pressure for a single day.
They don't carry your load.
They don't know your cost.
So why are you curving your path for their comfort?
You weren't built to be likeable.
You were built to break patterns.
To go further.
To create noise that doesn't fade.
The kind that echoes long after the crowd moves on.
So stop seeking consensus.
Start seeking consequence.
The kind that turns heads without asking for permission.

Stay Locked. Stay Cold. Stay Building.

The crowd will never understand.
It wasn't built to.
It thrives on sameness.
On safety.
On surface-level wins.
Show too much hunger, and they'll call it arrogance.
Show too much focus, and they'll call it obsession.
Show too much distance, and they'll say you've lost touch.
The reality is, you just stopped playing the crowd's game.

So let them label.

Let them misunderstand.
That's the tax you pay for refusing to live inside their limits.
You weren't made to fit the noise.
You were made to outgrow it and build something they can't ignore.

Put It On the Table.

Does this 'thought' hit home?
☐ Yes　☐ Not really

If yes, can you call yourself out and apply it?
☐ Yes　☐ Still hiding

If yes, what's one move you'll make to prove it's not just words?

....

....

Thought 24
Swaggajackers.

Everyone wants presence.
No one wants the scars.
Enter the Swaggajacker.
Props to my mate Umi for coining the term.
Once you hear it, and understand it, you'll start spotting them everywhere.
A Swaggajacker isn't real.
They're borrowing presence.
Walking like they've earned it.
Wearing confidence like a costume.
Scratch beneath the surface, and there's nothing underneath.
No grit. No substance. No truth.
Just show.
Just noise.
Just smoke.
Swagger they never sweated for.
Confidence on credit.

You Can Always Spot the Faker.

It's not hard.
The guy who trains once a week and rocks a Gold's Gym vest.
The girl reusing decade-old selfies, face flattened with filters.
The lad who gives it large in the pub but mysteriously vanishes when it kicks off.
The entrepreneur selling hustle but can't manage his inbox.
They dress the part.
Talk the part.

But they're allergic to real stakes.
Because it's easy to act tough when there's nothing to lose.

Swaggajackers are loud in safe rooms.
Bold when they're the sharpest voice in a dull circle.
But when pressure shows up - real, raw, non-negotiable pressure -
they ghost.
Because being fake takes zero courage.
It's like printing a degree you never studied for and hoping no one
checks.
But life will check.

Style Without Substance Always Cracks.

Pressure reveals everything.
You can fake composure in calm weather.
You can imitate someone else's confidence online.
But when life throws you heat, you either hold or fold.
Swaggajackers fold.
Quietly.
Quickly.
Because showmanship doesn't hold weight when reality starts
swinging.

Earned Energy Feels Different.

Real ones don't have to convince you.
They don't posture.
They carry presence not for show, but because it's built.
They don't shout because they don't need to.
They don't strut or peacock.
They've done the reps.
Taken the hits.
Failed.
And rebuilt.

You can feel it.
In the stare.
In the stillness.
In how they stand calm when things go sideways.
It's not vibes - it's the weight built from experience.
No bluff.
No panic.
No borrowed lines.
That's what earned feels like.
And once you've felt it, the fakes become obvious.

Real Isn't Trendy - It's Tiring.

Being real isn't sexy.
It's fucking exhausting.
It means showing up and holding standards when no one's watching.
It means choosing the harder road because you'd rather be solid than seen.
There's no shortcut to presence.
No 'big dick energy' can fake consistency.
You want depth?
You earn it in silence.
You build it in repetition.
You bleed for it without loading up IG Live.
Swaggajackers crave validation.
They want quick credit and curated clout.
They want the spotlight, but none of the scars.
But the real ones?
They're too focused on their own mission to chase approval.
They don't post the grind because they're actually in it.
No time to narrate - just build.
The twisted truth is that you pay either way.
Faking it costs as much as earning it, only with a worse return.
Swaggajacking drains you.
You're constantly maintaining the act.
Worried the mask will slip.
Trapped in a character that never fit in the first place.

That's a tax on your peace.
A weight you carry for validation that doesn't feed you.
But when you build it for real - when your confidence comes from scars, not stories - you stop pretending.
You don't flinch when questioned.
You don't shrink in heat.
You don't need permission to feel powerful because you've earned it, lived it, proved it.
So no, being real isn't flashy.
But it's free.
And it lasts.

Everyone Wants the Outcome. Few Want the Origin.

Everyone wants to look like they've made it.
But no one wants to show the making.
The pain.
The boredom.
The discipline that isn't sexy enough for stories.
Swaggajackers copy the outcome.
The car.
The attitude.
The lingo.
But they've skipped the actual road.
They'll mirror your moves but not your mindset.
They'll mimic your tone but not your trials.
That's why it rings hollow.
Because style without struggle is empty.
You can't steal someone's energy if you haven't lived their experience.
You can wear their words, but they won't land the same.
You can copy the walk, but not the weight they've carried.

The real ones didn't just arrive.
They bled for it.
They stood alone for seasons.
They walked through failure without flinching, and showed up again before anyone noticed.

Swaggajackers Want the Highlight Reel.

Your growth wasn't a montage - it was mess.
Repetition.
Unseen grit.
So don't be fooled by the gloss.
And don't let someone fake your frequency and then call it
'inspiration'.
Real doesn't copy.
It creates.
It doesn't echo.
It originates.
It doesn't need to be loud.
It just needs to be true.

Put It On the Table.

Does this 'thought' hit home?
☐ Yes   ☐ Not really

If yes, can you call yourself out and apply it?
☐ Yes   ☐ Still hiding

If yes, what's one move you'll make to prove it's not just words?

....

....

Thought 25
Old You, Old Limits.

You've outgrown yourself.
The version of you that carried you this far?
They've done their bit.
They fought the battles.
Took the risks.
Built the momentum.
You owe them gratitude, not permanence.
Because if you're serious about going further, you need to become someone else.
Not a shinier version or someone with more accolades.
But someone bolder.
More deliberate.
More aligned with the life you're now brave enough to imagine.

This isn't about improvement.
It's about transformation.
Because the life you're building won't fit the habits, mindset, or identity you're dragging from yesterday.

The Necessary Breakup.

Growth sounds noble in theory.
In practice, it feels like betrayal.
You're not just shedding bad habits.
You're letting go of parts of yourself that once kept you safe.
It's like retiring a loyal employee - perfect for the early days, but now they're holding the business back.
The comfort routines?

Gone.
The old self-talk?
Outdated.
The version of you who made excuses sound smart?
Redundant.
You'll second-guess yourself.
You'll feel disloyal.
But evolution doesn't wait for your feelings to catch up.
It demands change, not permission.
Letting go of your old self feels like a funeral - but it's the price of rebirth.
You're not burying the past to shame it.
You're burying it because you're ready to grow beyond it.

The Myth of Arrival.

Many treat success like a destination.
Hit the milestone, exhale, coast.
But real growth doesn't settle.
It knows comfort is often the first sign of decline.
Look at companies that straight up ruled their industries -
Nokia.
Kodak.
Blockbuster.
They didn't collapse from competition - they decayed from within.
They stopped adapting and started defending the past instead of inventing the future.
The market isn't sentimental and neither is life.
If you're not hungry, you're replaceable.
If you're not evolving, you're in decline - whether you admit it or not.

When What Helped You Now Hurts You.

One of the hardest pills to swallow...
Your strengths can become your weaknesses.

The discipline that got you through the early grind?
It might now be blinding you to smarter, more sustainable strategies.
The fire that made you relentless?
It could be burning you out because you never learned how to rest.
The mindset that helped you survive chaos?
It might now be sabotaging your peace.
Growth isn't just adding tools to your locker - it's knowing when to retire the ones that no longer serve.

Evolution Starts Internally.

People chase visible results - new income, new body, new status.
But transformation begins quietly.
With uncomfortable questions -
What am I doing that no longer reflects who I want to be?
Where am I choosing familiar over effective?
Who do I need to disappoint to stop betraying myself?
You need to really focus on alignment.
That starts with honesty - the kind that stings before it frees.
The answers are rarely pretty, but they're always honest.
And that honesty is the birthplace of reinvention.

The Collapse of Old Metrics.

As you evolve, the scorecard starts to prang out.
What used to light you up now leaves you cold.
The milestones that once felt like proof of progress feel strangely hollow. The hunger's changed, but you haven't caught up.
It messes with your head.
You start asking, "*What the fuck's wrong with me? Why doesn't this work anymore?*"
But it's not failure.
It's fracture - the breakdown of an identity that ran out of road.
You're not lazy.
You're not lost.

You've just outgrown your old fuel and you're still figuring out what the new engine runs on.
The real trap?
Trying to chase a bigger life with the same old motivations -
Approval.
Achievement.
Survival.
They built the foundation - but they can't build what comes next.
This next version of you?
They don't move from fear.
They move for alignment.
They don't perform to be seen.
They build to feel true.
And getting there will feel messy.
Like your internal compass is spinning.
Like nothing quite fits.
But that disorientation is evidence that you're shifting.
That means it's working.

Check Your Tools.

Here's your audit -
Are your routines built for maintenance or growth?
Maintenance keeps the lights on.
Growth builds something new.
If your habits feel efficient but uninspired, they're not serving your next level.
They're just keeping you busy.
Are your thoughts focused on preservation or possibility?
A mindset shaped in survival won't help you thrive.
It'll make you cautious when you need to be bold.
Are you living by default or by design?
When's the last time you questioned your systems - not just what you do, but why?
Default is easy.
Familiar.
But it's also where dreams go to die.

The version of you that got you here might still have momentum.
But momentum in the wrong direction is just drift.
Sometimes you're not stuck because you're failing - you're stuck because you're succeeding at things you've already outgrown.
Stop polishing what needs to be replaced.
You don't remodel a crumbling house if the foundation's fucked.
You rebuild with new tools, sharper focus, and a clearer blueprint that reflects who you've become.
Take inventory.
Not just of your habits, but of your identity.
Because if your tools are outdated, your results will be too.

Build the One Who'll Take You Further.

This next version of you?
They're not born from tweaks.
They're forged in clarity, courage, and reinvention.
They don't cling to what worked.
They build what's needed.
They don't react.
They lead.
They understand this -
The next level isn't a continuation - it's a reconfiguration.
So yes, thank the version of you who got you here.
But don't ask them to run the next race.
They were built for survival.
Now it's time to build for expansion.
Let go of the familiar to make space for the possible.
Evolve.
Boldly, deliberately, unapologetically.
Because the version of you that got you here?
They've done their job.
Now it's your turn to become the one who'll take you the rest of the way.

Put It On the Table.

Does this 'thought' hit home?
☐ Yes   ☐ Not really

If yes, can you call yourself out and apply it?
☐ Yes   ☐ Still hiding

If yes, what's one move you'll make to prove it's not just words?

....

....

Thought 26
Every "Yes" Is a "No" to Something Else.

Every time you say *"yes"*, something else dies.
Might be your time.
Might be your focus.
Might be the one damn hour you had to yourself all week.
But it dies.
Quietly.
Without a funeral.
And you're the one who pulled the trigger.

Most people don't clock the cost.
They just keep nodding their way into a life that doesn't fit.
Buried under favours, guilt, and shit they never wanted to do in the first place.

"Yes" is the Easiest Way to Lose Yourself.

People say *"yes"* to avoid friction.
To look good.
To stay liked.
The truth is - *"yes"* is a shortcut with a long hangover.
You say *"yes"* to be polite, now you're stuck in a meeting that's eating your soul.
You say *"yes"* to help out, now you're behind on your own grind.
You say *"yes"* because it feels easier, now you're exhausted, bitter, and no closer to what you actually want.

And for what?
You don't get extra points for being agreeable.
You just get used.

If You Don't Guard Your Time, No One Else Will.

You don't need to be booked out to feel burnt out.
All it takes is saying yes to the wrong shit, over and over, until your life's just noise.
People talk about time management like it's some neat little system.
Wrong.
It's warfare.
And the battleground is your inbox, your calendar, your DMs, your people-pleasing reflex.
Say yes to everything, and soon you're no longer choosing your life, you're just reacting to everyone else's script.
And the kicker?
You let this happen.

Saying No Is a Discipline. Train It.

Want clarity?
Say no.
Want freedom?
Say no faster.
Want peace?
Say no so often it starts to scare people.
It's not about being harsh.
It's about being real.
Your time isn't community property.
Your energy isn't on tap.
And your future isn't something to gamble on out of politeness.

Start here...
Don't answer questions right away.
Make space.

Even ten seconds of silence can snap you out of your old habits.
Ask yourself - *"If I say yes to this, what gets pushed off the cliff?"*
Don't just consider what you're agreeing to.
Look at what you're sacrificing.
Because the price of yes isn't written in ink.
It's written in the things that quietly disappear when you don't protect them.

The Life You Hate Is Built One Yes at a Time.

Nobody wakes up overwhelmed because of one big decision.
It's not an explosion - it's a slow leak.
You let one request slide in.
Then another.
Then another.
And before long, your day is packed with shit you didn't choose, for people you don't like, chasing outcomes you don't give two fucks about.
That's the price of the unfiltered yes.
If you're tired all the time, it's probably not your work ethic.
It's your boundaries.
And the longer you ignore your boundaries, the faster your life floods with regret.

You're Not a Bad Person for Protecting Your Sanity.

Want to keep your fire?
Protect your space like it's sacred.
That doesn't mean being a dickhead.
It means choosing your own mission over someone else's comfort.
It means saying -
"That's not a priority right now."
"I'm not available for that."
"I don't do that anymore."
No drama.
No drawn-out excuse.

Just clean lines.
Because the version of you that gets shit done, lives sharp, and feels alive - needs room to breathe.
And yes is a chokehold if you're not careful.

"No" Is How You Stay Dangerous.

You want to stay useful to your goals?
Stop being so available.
Stop filling your calendar with pointless tasks out of guilt.
Stop grabbing your ankles to support people who drain you.
Stop saying "yes" to things that make you resentful five minutes later.
Every "no" is a defence of your mission.
Every "no" is a sharpening of your focus.
Every "no" is a step closer to being the person who actually lives how they talk.
Feeling self-conscious about people calling you - 'The No Guy'?
Grow up - people will be fine.
The world won't crumble because you chose yourself.

Nobody Respects What You Don't Protect.

People don't take advantage of your time because they're evil.
They do it because you let them.
So if your days feel hijacked, ask yourself -
"When did I open the door?"
"When did I nod instead of push back?"
"When did I smile through the resentment and call it 'being nice'?"
The hardest truth?
You teach people how to treat you.
Not with words, but with what you tolerate.
You want to change the dynamic?
Start saying "no".
Loudly.
Early.
Without the guilt-soaked cushion.

Make Every "Yes" Count.

Here's the rule...
If it doesn't move you forward, feed your spirit, or strengthen your cause - it's a "no".
You don't have unlimited bandwidth.
You don't have endless patience.
And you sure as hell don't have time to waste.
So treat your "yes" like it's sacred.
Like it's something rare.
Like it builds your future one brilliant brick at a time.

Put It On the Table.

Does this 'thought' hit home?
☐ Yes　☐ Not really

If yes, can you call yourself out and apply it?
☐ Yes　☐ Still hiding

If yes, what's one move you'll make to prove it's not just words?

....

....

Part 4

MASTER THE MIND

Thought 27
Don't Be Scared Homie.

I don't know why we exist.
I don't know how we got here.
But I do know one thing for certain - we are all going to die.

Sorry for the harsh opener.
While I'm at it - Santa isn't real, the world isn't flat, and any bloke
wearing a scarf with a T-shirt indoors is, objectively, a cunt.
Now that we've stripped away the fairytales, let's talk reality.
If we know the ending is death - no refunds, no replays - it baffles me
how many people are happy to live anything but a full life.
They sleepwalk through decades.
They play it safe until the final whistle.
The finish line's coming whether you sprint, crawl, or just stand there
scrolling.
What's the fucking point if you never really showed up?

Life Is a Chocolate Bar.

Life is like a box of chocolates…
You hand me that box and I'm eating them all.
One sitting.
No hesitation.
Now imagine this - I'm going to take six out of the eight chocolates,
roll them in shit, and then eat them…
You'd look at me like I'd lost my fucking mind.
And you'd be right.
But people do this every single day, metaphorically.
They take the best parts of their life - their time, their talent, their

energy - and contaminate them with fear.
They rationalise it.
They wrap it up in logic.
In - "*good sense*".
They call it - "being realistic".
They tell themselves they're being responsible, when really they're just choosing beige over colour, comfort over courage, and silence over truth.
They wear that choice like it's a medal.
Like shrinking yourself is noble.
Like settling is maturity.
They think it's what you're supposed to do.

Fear Shrinks the Window.

We get roughly 80 years if we're lucky.
That's our window of opportunity.
And fear?
Fear's job is to make that window smaller.
Bit by bit.
It's the voice that whispers -
"*Be safe.*"
"*Don't stand out.*"
"*Don't take the risk.*"
"*Stay comfortable.*"
Fear tells you not to smile at strangers.
Not to speak too loudly.
Not to say what you really think.
Not to dream bigger than the people around you.
It clips your wings until you're just a cardboard cut-out of the human you were meant to be.
Fear doesn't want you dead - it just wants you muted.

The Big Three Fears.

Most fear boils down to three things -

Money, security, relationships.
Those three wear different costumes, but it's always the same play.
Fear of not having enough.
Fear of losing what you have.
Fear of being left behind.
And yeah, they're important.
Money pays the bills.
Security helps you sleep at night.
Love keeps you human.
But when those fears start running the show?
When they dictate your every move?
You're not living. You're surviving.
You're caged in a comfort zone so padded, it might as well be a coffin.
That's when your dreams start to die.
That's when your spirit fades like a shit tattoo.
That's when you become a spectator in your own damn life.

Fuck Fear.

Let me be clear…
I'm not projecting some 'big dick energy' persona.
I don't think I'm invincible.
I just manage the conversation happening inside my own head.
That's all.
Fear still talks.
I just don't hand it the microphone.
A master of fear doesn't eliminate it - they study it.
They outwit it.
They edit the interior monologue.
You don't need to be fearless, you need to be fluent in fear.
Speak its language, know its lies.
Then act anyway.
That's how you go from victim to warrior.
From complainer to creator.
From spectator to fucking legend.

Fear Loves a Microphone.

Give fear airtime and watch it hijack your whole setlist.
You start scanning rooms for threats instead of opportunities.
You rehearse worst-case scenarios until they become reality in your head.
You have imaginary arguments that drain real energy.
You start backpedalling before you've even moved forward.
And the worst bit?
You think it's smart.
You think you're just being careful.
You think you're being mature.
But you're not.
You're being held hostage by a voice that's full of shit.

That fear you felt?
It becomes fact in your mind.
Not just a possibility, a certainty.
And so you don't try.
You don't risk.
You don't speak.
You just exist.
Your chocolate tastes like shit - and you chose it.

Flip the Script.

What if fear isn't the enemy?
What if fear is the signal you're getting close to something important?
Fear doesn't bother showing up for the trivial shit.
It reserves its energy for the moments that count before greatness.
Before change.
Before truth that might actually change your trajectory.
Fear is the bouncer outside the club where your best life's playing.
It stands there, arms folded, sizing you up.
Your job isn't to punch it in the face.
Your job is to nod, show ID, and walk in shoulders back.
The trick isn't to silence fear - you won't.

Fear is loud.
Fear is rude.
Fear will sit in the back seat and heckle you the whole way.
Your move is to drive anyway.
Hands on the wheel.
Eyes forward.
Let fear be the passenger, not the pilot.

There are no hidden secrets here.
You just show up.
Say the thing.
Launch the project.
Ask the question.
Book the ticket.
Do it scared.
Fear can come along for the ride, but it doesn't get to drive.

Leave Nothing in the Tank.

When death knocks, I'm not answering the door with fuel in the tank.
I want to meet him like a Peperami wrapper - torn to bits, greasy, and completely fucking empty.
No "*untapped potential.*"
No "*someday.*"
No holding back.
No clean fingernails.

Too many people tiptoe toward the grave, worried about what might go wrong while life flies past.
I'd rather sprint toward it battered, bruised, proud of every scar I earned along the way.
The goal was never to survive life, it was to spend it.
All of it.
Loudly.
Boldly.
Recklessly if necessary.

George Bernard Shaw nailed it when he said -
"Life is no 'brief candle' for me. It is a sort of splendid torch which I have got hold of for the moment, and I want to make it burn as brightly as possible before handing it on to future generations."
That's the energy.
Not a flicker.
Not a polite glow.
A fireball.
So burn it all.
Burn with purpose.
Burn with love.
Burn with rage, laughter, tears, whatever you've got.
And when it's over?
Let them say, *"They didn't waste a single fucking spark."*
Don't be scared homie. Be unstoppable.

Put It On the Table.

Does this 'thought' hit home?
☐ Yes ☐ Not really

If yes, can you call yourself out and apply it?
☐ Yes ☐ Still hiding

If yes, what's one move you'll make to prove it's not just words?

....

....

Thought 28
You've Only Got Ten Coins.

Imagine your life runs on currency.
But not pounds, dollars, or crypto.
Coins.
Ten of them.
That's it.
Each coin is your time.
Your energy.
Your focus.
Your daily bandwidth to give a fuck.

You don't get bonus coins for being passionate.
You don't get rollover coins for hustling extra hard.
It doesn't matter if you're a wizard or a wild pig - you get ten.
And every single thing you commit to - career, relationship, hobby,
health, family, healing, side hustle - it all costs coins.
Spend wisely.

Where Are Your Coins Going?

This isn't about guilt.
This isn't about hustle culture.
This is about clarity.

Your ten coins are already being spent, whether you notice or not.
Some are flying out of your pocket on autopilot.
Some are buried in shit that looks productive but drains you without
moving forward.

Some are going to people who wouldn't piss on you if you were on fire.
And sometimes?
You're tossing coins into the abyss and calling it ambition.
This isn't about shame.
It's about asking -
"Where the fuck are my coins going?
And is it worth the cost?"

The Bath Salt Moment.

Last year I had this business idea.
Bath salts for men.
Stay with me...
It sounds ridiculous, I know, but I could see it smashing the market to pieces.
The branding was sharp.
The concept was tight.
I found a supplier.
Negotiated terms.
I was one click away from ordering a tonne (literally) of Himalayan pink.
But just before I hit 'go', I paused...
Not because I didn't believe in the idea - I still do.
But because I did a coin check.

Where would the coins come from?
Would I take them from my daughter?
From my health?
From the business I've already built?
Because something else always has to pay.
That's the law of the ten coins.

So I checked my ego and walked away.
Not because it was a bad idea, but because I wasn't willing to reshuffle my coins to make it work.
And that decision?

That was self-respect.

You Can Do Anything, But Not Everything.

Social media's full of bullshit.
"Grind 24/7."
"Build an empire."
"Start five side hustles before breakfast."
Cool.
And when are you seeing your kids mate?
When are you sleeping?
When are you just being instead of always doing?
This culture convinced us we can juggle a hundred priorities with no trade-offs.
That we can balance it all like some kind of superhuman octopus.

But balance?
Balance is a scam.
You don't balance everything.
You choose what to carry and what to drop.
That means accepting some things will not get your best right now.
Not because you're lazy, but because you're smart enough to pick your battles.

The Trade-Off Test.

Want to start something new?
A business?
A relationship?
A fitness plan?
A hobby?
Good.
But first ask -
Which coin is this coming from?
Who or what gets less of me if this gets more?
Am I okay with that?

If you can't answer clearly, you're not making a smart decision.
You're en route to making a fucking mess.

Coins and Crisis.

Here's the part no one tells you - crisis spends your coins for you.
Grief.
Burnout.
Divorce.
Illness.
Debt.
When life smacks you in the mouth, it hijacks your wallet.
Suddenly, you've lost three coins just trying to function.
You've got nothing left for goals or growth or even socialising.
And if you don't adjust your spending?
You'll snap.

This is where most people go wrong.
They pretend their coin count hasn't changed.
They try to keep up the same routine, same grind, same face.
And then they wonder why they're falling apart.
Sometimes the bravest move isn't pushing harder.
It's downsizing your life to match your reality.
That's not quitting.
That's surviving with strategy.

Don't Outsource Your Coins.

If you don't consciously choose where your ten coins go, someone
else will.
Your boss will.
Your inbox will.
Your phone will.
Your insecurities will.
And one day, you'll wake up five years deep in a life that doesn't fit,
and wonder why you feel hollow.

That's the price of passive coin-spending.
If you don't set your values and guard your priorities, you become a vending machine for other people's bullshit.
And nothing drains you faster than coins spent out of guilt and obligation.

Your Coins, Your Call.

I don't care how you spend your ten coins.
Want to spend all ten building an empire?
Go for it.
Want to spend seven on your kids, and three making protein snacks for dogs with separation anxiety?
Beautiful.
There's no 'right' way to spend them, there's just your way, lived on purpose.
But you owe it to yourself to know where your coins are going, why they're going there, and whether it's still worth it.
If something's changed?
Redistribute.
Realign.
Restructure.
Because the second you start spending your coins with intention, you stop living out of guilt, habit, or fear.
And you start living like someone who owns their fucking life.

Put It On the Table.

Does this 'thought' hit home?
☐ Yes   ☐ Not really

If yes, can you call yourself out and apply it?
☐ Yes   ☐ Still hiding

If yes, what's one move you'll make to prove it's not just words?

....

....

Thought 29
Peace Is the Most Hardcore Thing You Can Chase.

You think being loud makes you powerful?
That chaos means you're alive?
That adrenaline equals purpose?
Wrong.
That's just survival mode disguised as ambition.
It's noise.
It's ego.
It's fear wearing a lion's face.
You want to know what's really hard?
Getting your mind quiet.
Living without drama.
Sitting in your own company without scrambling for a screen, a fight, or a fix.
That's real fucking power.
Real power doesn't explode.
It contains.
It measures.
It chooses its moments.

I Used to Think Peace Was for the Weak.

I thought calm meant quitting.
That peace was what people settled for when they stopped striving.

But I was wrong.
Sometimes the most frantic movement is just someone outrunning themselves.
I chased the next win like it would finally shut the voices up.
The next problem like solving it would prove I mattered.
But the truth?
I was addicted to chaos because it distracted me from looking in the mirror.
Stillness would've meant facing myself.
And back then, that was the scariest thing in the world.

The Real Battlefield Is Between Your Ears.

We walk through life thinking we're fighting the system.
Our past.
Our enemies.
But most people aren't in a fight with the outside world.
They're shadowboxing their own insecurities.
The real war is with the thoughts that whisper -
"You're only as valuable as your output."
"Keep running, or you'll fall apart."
"Rest is for the weak."
That isn't drive.
It's fear with a work ethic.
Peace is the weapon that disarms that bullshit.
But it requires a kind of inner strength that never makes it onto your CV.
There's no medal for choosing peace.
No crowd claps when you walk away instead of throwing a punch.
And that's the headline - if you need a crowd to validate your win, you're not really free.
Freedom is knowing you can fight and still deciding you don't need to.
It's recognising that the loudest battles are sometimes just ego in costume.
It's winning without witnesses.
Because when you can lay your weapons down without feeling smaller?

That's when you've already won.

Stillness Isn't Stagnation.

Stillness isn't giving up.
It's gearing up.
It's what happens when you trust your foundation enough to wait for the right moment instead of chasing every shiny thing.
The person who can pause, hold their ground, and not flinch - that's the real threat.
Not the loudest in the room, but the one who's fully present and doesn't need to be seen.
When you stop performing and start observing, the whole game changes.
You stop getting baited into battles that don't matter.
You stop reacting and start choosing.
Stillness is a flex most people don't understand.

Learn to Be Unshakeable.

Anyone can yell.
Anyone can rage.
That's not dominance, that's desperation.
The apex player?
The one who can hold their gaze steady and unreadable while chaos swings for their head.
They don't flinch because they've already fought - and won - the war within.
They don't bark orders or beg for validation because their power isn't performative.
It's rooted.
And rooted people are dangerous.
Not because they'll come at you, but because you can't move them.
Not with praise.
Not with pressure.
Not with fear.

Stop Wrestling Ghosts.

There's a kind of peace that comes when you realise not every conflict needs your presence.
Not every provocation is an invitation.
I used to treat every disagreement like it was a test of my worth.
Like if I didn't respond, I'd lose something.
Now I see it differently.
If someone's committed to misunderstanding you, clarity won't help.
And logic won't either.
Your truth will get twisted.
Sometimes the only message they can't manipulate is your absence.
So walk away - not from fear, but from knowing exactly what staying will cost you.

Burn Without Burning Out.

Peace doesn't mean complacency.
It doesn't mean shrinking.
It means fuelling your fire with purpose, not panic.
You can still go all in.
Still hunt the throne.
Still crush the competition.
But you're doing it from a place of wholeness, not emptiness.
That's the shift.
You stop trying to earn your worth through exhaustion - stop proving your power through pain.
You build.
You rest.
You rise.
You say no.
You become selective about what gets your fire.
Because not everything deserves to be burned for.

Peace Doesn't Mean Passive. It Means Planted.

There's a kind of movement that looks like stillness from the outside but is unstoppable from within.
You're not running anymore.
You're rooted.
You're not hustling for scraps of approval.
You know your value.
You're not everywhere because you've learned that presence beats performance.
That kind of peace is not a pause - it's a strategy.
It's how you outlast, outgrow, and outshine.

Peace Isn't a Vibe. It's an Operating System.

Peace isn't an aesthetic.
It's not soft tones and soft talk.
It's hard lines.
Non-negotiables.
Boundaries you don't explain.
It's discipline over impulse.
Purpose over performance.
It's knowing when to speak and when to stay silent.
When to walk and when to stay planted.
When to burn and when to breathe.
Most people don't have that operating system - because they've never sat still long enough to install it.

Hold the Line.

You want to know what separates the ones who build legacies from the ones who burn out?
The line.
The line they refuse to cross, even when they're provoked, tempted, or doubted.
Peace isn't just calm - it's control.

Of your time.
Your attention.
Your energy.
You don't throw that away for cheap applause.
You don't spend it on small minds.
You hold the fucking line.
Because real power isn't about how loud you roar.
It's in how deeply you're rooted when the storm comes.
And if you've done the work?
That storm doesn't stand a chance.

Put It On the Table.

Does this 'thought' hit home?
☐ Yes   ☐ Not really

If yes, can you call yourself out and apply it?
☐ Yes   ☐ Still hiding

If yes, what's one move you'll make to prove it's not just words?

....

....

Thought 30
Venting Isn't Healing, It's Hiding.

Talking about it isn't the same as changing it.
There's a difference between letting it out and letting it rule you.
You can scream into the void, write twelve paragraphs of your story, cry on your best mate's couch, and still be neck-deep in the same wreckage you started with.
Venting feels good.
You blow off steam.
You rant to your partner.
You make a dramatic *"just being real"* post online, thinking vulnerability equals transformation.
However, most of the time venting is not healing.
It's just bleeding in public and calling it progress.
You haven't stitched the wound - you've just flung blood on the walls and asked people to admire the splatter.

Pain Doesn't Disappear Just Because You Say It Out Loud.

This culture has glorified emotional exposure.
Every breakdown gets a highlight reel.
Oversharing is seen as courage when sometimes it's just avoidance with a better caption.
Yes - speak your truth.
Yes - own your story.
But don't confuse that with building a better one.
Pain doesn't shrink when it's broadcasted.

It grows.
It multiplies when echoed through other people's reactions.
You say it out loud, and for five minutes, you feel seen.
But being seen isn't the same as being better.

We've made confession the finish line, when it's barely the starting block.
The real graft begins after the talking stops.
After the pity fades.
After the comments dry up.
You can tell your trauma story to a thousand people, but it still won't unpick your patterns.
Healing is ugly, lonely, and unrewarded.
It's not Instagrammable.
It's you sweating through the silence, rewiring the part of your brain that flinches at love or trust.
True healing isn't public theatre.
It's the unposted moments where you sit with the ache, face it, and change something real.
Because pain shared for attention feeds the wound.
But pain faced in private?
That's the stuff that closes it.

Venting Feels Like Movement But It's a Loop.

It tricks you.
You get a buzz from being raw, from being seen.
You feel lighter.
Like you've done something.
And that's the trap.
It's an emotional treadmill.
You're running full tilt, but you never leave the same square of pain.
You vent.
You get comfort.
You feel momentarily strong - and then you spiral.
Validation becomes your morphine.
You need people to keep nodding, keep caring, keep engaging with

your chaos.
Suddenly, you're not recovering.
You're performing.
You become the struggle.
Your darkness is your calling card.
You decorate your dysfunction with quotes about resilience and expect applause for enduring what you refuse to escape.

There's a Time for Talking and a Time for Doing.

Speaking up matters.
Keeping everything bottled up will rot you from the inside.
But speaking alone won't save you.
There comes a point where you've got to shut your mouth and move your feet.
Cry if you need to, but cry while doing something different.
Rage, but rage with direction.
Pain has energy.
Use it to fuel the climb, not to throw another tantrum at the bottom of the mountain.
Progress is a verb.
It's measured in changed choices, not poetic captions.
If the only muscle you've built is the one that writes status updates, you're not healing - you're lost in the feedback loop and calling it clarity.

You Can't Heal in the Same Room You Broke In.

Some people stay broken because it's familiar.
They know the lines.
They've rehearsed the identity.
They're addicted to the sympathy it buys.
They say they want growth, but what they really want is applause without effort.
So they 'process'.
They 'unpack'.

They go to therapy, talk in circles for a decade, but never take a different step.
Because real healing?
That shit costs.
It'll strip your ego.
It demands your pride.
It asks you to forgive people who will never make it right.
Healing means you stop milking your wounds for significance.
It means you walk away from being 'the hurt one' and start becoming 'the responsible one'.

Venting Isn't Evil, It's Just a Poor Substitution.

Venting has its place.
There's value in blowing the top off before you explode.
There's wisdom in not letting emotions rot in silence.
But if venting is your main strategy, you've chosen short-term relief over long-term repair.
You wouldn't spit in your engine and call it maintenance - so stop thinking emotional vomit counts as inner work.
Sometimes the most radical thing you can do is say nothing and act.
Change your routine.
Burn the excuses.
Shut up and get brutal with your own patterns.
The hard truth? Nobody's coming to rescue you from your own repetition.
No post.
No comment.
No hug.
That's all borrowed power.
And borrowed power runs out.

The High of Being Heard Is Cheap.

Society has an addiction to being consoled.
To being witnessed.

You want someone to say - *"That must be so hard."*
But what you need is someone who says - *"Now what?"*
The people who actually change are the ones who let their pain embarrass them into action.
They get tired of repeating themselves.
Sick of hearing their own sob story.
They stop performing grief and start auditing their daily choices.
They walk into the fire with purpose, not just a selfie.

Let It Burn But Don't Live There.

Feel your feelings.
Scream into the wind if that's what it takes to clear the static.
But don't build a house in the storm and call it home.
Let the mother fucker burn.
Burn mother fucker, burn…
But don't sit there roasting marshmallows in your own despair.
Use the flame.
Forge something.
Sharpen yourself on it.
Venting is the prelude not the plot.
You don't win just because you said it.
You win because you did something after saying it.

Own It or Loop It.

Every moment you vent without evolving, you're reinforcing the cage.
And cages - even golden ones - still keep you stuck.
This isn't about silencing yourself, it's about redirecting your power.
Not just noise, but impact.
Not just catharsis, but conversion.
You're allowed to be in pain.
You're not allowed to make it your throne.

Healing Starts Where Venting Stops.

So go ahead.
Feel it.
Name it.
But then walk into the silence that follows and do the fucking work.
The next version of you isn't found in another outburst.
It's built in the dark, with grit, with choices, with patterns you don't post about.
Say less.
Move more.
And if you're serious about healing, stop venting and start building.

Put It On the Table.

Does this 'thought' hit home?
☐ Yes ☐ Not really

If yes, can you call yourself out and apply it?
☐ Yes ☐ Still hiding

If yes, what's one move you'll make to prove it's not just words?

....

....

Thought 31
The Real You Only Shows Up When It's Ugly

Everyone's got a highlight reel.
Photoshopped smiles.
Curated wins.
Clean and tidy stories.
That's who we think we are and who we want others to believe we are.
The neat little version.
Easy on the eyes.
Easy to digest.
But the real version of you?
The one that counts?
That one only shows up when everything is all fucked up.

Pain Strips Off the Mask.

Want to know who you really are?
Don't look when life's good.
That version's too polished, too staged, too temporary to be trusted.
Look at yourself when it's dark, confusing, heavy.
When everything's cracked and no one's watching.
When the phone rings and it's bad news, again.
When your body gives out mid-session and you're gasping for more than air.
When someone you love says - *"You've changed,"* and it's not a compliment.
When you're running in the pissing rain, soaked to the bone, and everything screams to stop.

That's when the real you strolls in.
Not dressed up.
Not clean.
Just bare knuckle presence.

You Don't Meet Yourself in Comfort.

Comfort is where the masks thrive.
From comfort, you can bluff.
Perform.
Stay soft without challenge.
But out in the grit, in the fire - that's where you meet yourself.
At mile 20 of a marathon when your legs are toast and your lungs feel like sandpaper.
When you're called out in front of your peers and your instinct is to rage or retreat.
When you're not picked, not praised, not even seen.
That's your DNA.
The raw file.
No gloss.
No lies.
Just what you're really made of.
You only meet that version when everything else breaks.
And when they show up?
They bring answers.
Not the ones you give when you're safe.
The ones that crawl out from the pit of your gut when it's desperate and there's nowhere left to run.
That's when the truth stands up.
But brace yourself - you might not like the answer.

Adversity Isn't a Test, It's a Reveal.

People say hard times 'test' you.
Wrong.
They don't test - they show.

They show your real limits.
What you run toward, what you run from.
Whether your values are unshakable or just wallpaper you slapped up to look good.
And in the real world, you find out fast.
Do you fight or freeze?
Hold the line or crumble?
Bounce or break?
And this isn't bad.
It's gold.
Because now you've got data.
No guesswork.
Just you.
Once you've seen it, you can't unsee it.
You can run or you can build from it.
The smart ones build.
They take what pain exposed and turn it into armour.

Strength Looks Like Staying.

We talk a lot about breaking through.
About pushing past the pain.
But what about staying in it?
Real strength isn't just about rising.
It's about staying.
Staying when it's uncomfortable.
When everything in you is begging to bail.
When you've seen the exit sign a hundred times and your whole body aches for the relief of walking away.
And it would be easier - so much easier - to walk.
But you don't.
You stay.
That's a different kind of hard.
Not the heroic, movie-scene hard where you charge into battle and win in ten minutes.
Rather the kind where you sit among the wreckage and whisper -
"Alright... I'm not done yet."

Because sometimes growth isn't a sprint.
It's a slow grind.
It's getting up without the promise of a breakthrough.
It's having the same brutal conversation with yourself for the fiftieth time and still showing up to get it right.
It's resisting the knee-jerk to run when the weight gets too real.
People think strength is loud.
It's not.
Sometimes it's just breathing through the storm.
Sometimes it's biting your tongue when you really want to unload.
Sometimes it's keeping your heart open when every scar is telling you to slam the gates shut.
Staying looks like answering the phone even when you're dreading the voice on the other end.
It looks like getting up again when yesterday nearly killed you.
Staying makes you dangerous.
In that quietly unshakeable - *"I've been through hell and kept standing"* kind of way.
The kind of dangerous that doesn't bluff.
Doesn't rattle.
Doesn't need to prove anything.
Because once you've learned how to stay through the storm, you stop fearing it.
You stop giving your power away to discomfort.
You stop needing the world to be easy just so you can function.
You become the one who can hold the line.

That's where the real edge is forged.
That's where staying becomes strength.
Not because it's pretty.
Not because it's heroic.
But because you did it anyway.

The Ugly Moments Are the Honest Ones.

You can lie to the world.

Hell, you can even lie to yourself.
But when you're alone, exhausted, and nothing's going to plan - truth walks in and locks the door.
Ugly moments clean the lens.
Strip ego.
Demand honesty.
And honesty isn't always pretty.
But it's always solid.
Always useful.
It's the raw material you can actually build from.
If you're chasing a version of yourself that never bleeds, never breaks, never doubts - you're not chasing strength.
You're chasing a fucking cartoon.
Real strength stumbles before it stands.
It cries in the shower, then shows up anyway.
It admits the fear, then faces it with shaking hands.
The world doesn't need your flawless mask.
It needs the version of you that stayed when every cell screamed -
"*Leave!*"
Because that's the version that's real.
That's the version that lasts.

Stop Avoiding the Mirror.

Everyone wants growth.
Few want self-awareness.
It's easier to post a quote than admit you're fragile.
Easier to keep grinding than to ask - "*Am I actually okay?*"
The strongest people I know have all broken.
And they didn't tape it up with hustle quotes.
They rebuilt.
Brick by brick.
Honest.
Different.
Stronger.

They didn't avoid the cracked mirror.
They stared into it until something real stared back.
And when it did?
They owned it.

You want real power?
Start there.
In the mirror.
Even if it's cracked.
Especially if it's cracked.

Your Darkness Has a Name. It's You.

The ugly moments don't create a new you.
They introduce you to the one who's been waiting all along.
That voice that doesn't quit.
That instinct that fights through pain.
That spirit that refuses to stay down.
That's not a new you - it's the OG.
The one that doesn't give a fuck about comfort zones or curated perfection.
You don't need to chase that version.
You just need to let life strip the soft, fake layers off until only the real remains.
The real you only shows up when it's ugly.
So if it's ugly right now?
Lean in.
That's where the gold lives.
That's where the bullshit burns off and the bones show.
That's where you stop being a highlight reel and start being undeniable.

Put It On the Table.

Does this 'thought' hit home?
☐ Yes   ☐ Not really

If yes, can you call yourself out and apply it?
☐ Yes   ☐ Still hiding

If yes, what's one move you'll make to prove it's not just words?

....

....

Thought 32
Guard the Gate.

Let me tell you something that'll change the way you think -
Your mind is a gate.
And every thought, message, opinion, notification, and headline is
trying to get through it.
Most people leave that gate wide open.
No filter.
No lock.
No awareness.
They let any old noise walk in, kick its shoes off, and dump shit on the
carpet.
And then they scratch their heads, wondering why they're anxious.
Why they can't focus.
Why they never feel like they're making progress.
The truth is they don't have a discipline problem - they've got a
boundary problem.
They never learned to guard the gate.
They never asked - *"Does this deserve space in my head?"*
If they had, most of that noise would've been bounced at the door
before it even got close.

Focus Is the Rarest Resource You Have.

You think time is your most valuable resource?
Wrong.
Focus is the fucking currency.
Time without focus?
Useless.

You can sit in front of your laptop for five hours and get nothing done, because you've let every pointless distraction flood in and occupy space in your head.
Focus is how you direct your energy.
And energy is how you build, move, grow, and win.
Lose focus, and you lose power.
People yap about *"hustling harder,"* but skip the part where their attention is fractured into a thousand pieces.
You can't dominate your day if you're mentally scattered before breakfast.
You can't lead, build, or love properly if you're splitting your focus across bullshit inputs.
Want to level up?
Start with what you're letting in.

The World Is Coming for Your Attention.

Every app.
Every platform.
Every ad.
Every headline.
They're all engineered to hijack your brain.
Plot twist - I'm one of the architects of your distraction.
I work in digital advertising.
I know exactly how this game is played because I play it.
Professionally.
My job is to design content that cuts through the noise, interrupts your scroll, and burrows into your head.
When I run a campaign for a client, I'm not coming for your wallet straight away.
That's amateur hour.
I'm coming for your attention.
Because attention is the gateway drug.
It's the real currency.
If I can get your eyes for three seconds, I can buy another ten.
And if I get ten, I can start changing how you think, what you value, even how you feel about yourself.

Once I've got that?
Game over.
You're not just seeing my ad.
You're playing my game.

And that game?
It's everywhere.
It's not just ads.
It's every swipe, every scroll, every dopamine-dripping notification designed to manipulate your thoughts.
The whole system is rigged to steal your attention and sell it back to you as anxiety.
And you think you're just *"checking your phone for a second"*?
Wrong.
You're throwing open the fucking gate.
Letting in comparison.
The rage.
The insecurity.
The highlight reels, the clickbait, and the *"you should be doing more"* propaganda.
And it doesn't leave quietly.
It lingers.
It eats into your mental energy before you've even had your first coffee.
You don't feel tired because you worked hard, you feel tired because your brain's been under siege since the moment you woke up.
And that exhaustion?
That fog?
That's the cost of an unguarded gate.

Be Brutal With Access.

Not just with your phone.
With people.
With opinions.
With media.
With noise.

Most of it is mental junk food.
Tastes good.
Feels easy.
Leaves you bloated and unfocused.
You've got to start treating your mind like premium real estate.
Not everything gets a key.
You wouldn't let a stranger dump rubbish in your house.
So why let them do it in your mind?
Being 'open' isn't always virtuous.
Sometimes it's just weak boundaries pretending to be tolerance.
You don't have to explain why you don't want to engage.
You don't need to justify silence.
Clarity is a by-product of curation.
Get selective.

You Don't Need to Know Everything, You Need to Know Yourself.

Here's the trap - we've sold ourselves on being 'informed' by swallowing every perspective, argument, opinion, trend, disaster, and debate.
The truth is you don't need to consume everything - you need to be intentional.
You don't need to know what everyone's saying - you need to know what you believe.

Clarity doesn't come from more input.
It comes from less noise.
You're not a hard drive - you're a human.
And the more mental clutter you carry, the less bandwidth you've got for what matters.
If you want to move clean, think clean.
And thinking clean starts by closing the gate to shit that doesn't belong.

How I Guard My Gate.

People think discipline is just about lifting weights and saying no to cake.
Wrong.
Discipline is mental hygiene.
Here's what I do...
I limit what comes into my phone.
No notifications unless they're critical.
Everything else?
Muted.
I mute or block anything that doesn't serve my mission.
I don't need a digital soap opera in my pocket.
I unsubscribe from noise.
If the content's not building me, I don't care how entertaining it is.
It's gone.
I keep my circle tight.
No passive aggressive energy thieves.
No one who makes me question my fire.
I protect my morning like it's sacred.
First 90 minutes?
Mine.
No input.
Only output.
When I feel scattered, I pull back.
I pause.
I sharpen the sword.
No guilt.

It looks 'cold' when I write down my process and see it in black and white.
But it's not cold - it's focus.
Because if I don't guard the gate, I can't lead.
Can't build.
Can't be present for the people who actually matter.

You Are the Guard.

You don't need to meditate more.
You don't need another self-help book.
You need to wake up to what you're letting into your life - and then start defending your mind like your future depends on it.
Every day you leave the gate unguarded, you let distractions in that dilute your mission.
That means goals you never hit.
Ideas you never build.
Relationships you never deepen.
Because you were too mentally compromised to go all in.
So be ruthless.
Be selective.
Be clear.
You are the gatekeeper.
Not everything gets in.
And not everything deserves to.

Let the wrong thing in and it'll cost you peace, progress, and power.
But if you learn to say no?
If you protect the gate with intention and force?
You'll move like someone with clarity.
With presence.
With purpose.
That's what focus feels like.
Quiet.
Clean.
And once you've tasted that, chaos will feel disgusting.
Guard the gate.
Because if you don't?
Someone else will walk through it - and write your story for you.

Put It On the Table.

Does this 'thought' hit home?
☐ Yes   ☐ Not really

If yes, can you call yourself out and apply it?
☐ Yes   ☐ Still hiding

If yes, what's one move you'll make to prove it's not just words?

....

....

Thought 33
Joy Is a Middle Finger to the System.

Burnout is the currency of modern success.
Everyone's hustling.
Grinding.
Bleeding for the badge of 'busy'.
We wear exhaustion like it's proof we're doing something meaningful.
You know what that is?..

Fucking tragic.

When did being miserable become a flex?
When did we decide that self-destruction was the ticket to self-respect?
What about joy?
Joy isn't soft.
It's not cotton-wool bullshit for the weak.
Joy is the middle finger you throw up to a culture that told you you're only worthy when you're suffering.

The System Wants You Exhausted.

Not tired - fucking exhausted.
So drained you can't think straight.
So jacked on stimulants and deadlines that you forget you're a human, not a cog in someone else's machine.
It wants you glued to your screen, comparing yourself to strangers.

It wants you chasing gold stars, likes, promotions, praise from people who'd forget your name if you stopped performing.
It wants you hooked on caffeine, stress, and shame.
Why?
Because if you're too tired to think, you're easy to control.
You'll follow the script.
You'll buy more shit.
You'll stress more.
You'll keep scrolling, keep consuming, keep obeying.
And you won't stop long enough to ask the only question that matters
- *"Am I actually living a life I want?"*
That's the question they're scared of.
Because once you ask that, the whole house of cards starts to shake.
So when you choose joy - raw, loud, unfiltered - you're not opting out.
You're fighting back.
You're saying -
"I don't need to hate my life to prove I'm working hard."
"I'm not sacrificing my peace to make someone else rich."
"I'm not available for the worship of burnout anymore."

Joy Is a Weapon. Use It.

Laughing when life's heavy?
That's not ignorance.
That's alchemy.
It's transmutation.
It's grabbing pain by the throat and saying - *"You don't get to own all of me."*
Smiling in traffic jams.
Dancing in your kitchen.
Playing with your kid like the world isn't burning down around you.
That's strength with glitter on.
That's resistance without the scream.
Fun isn't frivolous, it's fuel.
It recharges the battery discipline runs on.
It's the oxygen for grit and the spark for resilience.
It reminds you that you're living, not a machine.

And don't get it twisted, you can be gritty and still enjoy your life. You can chase goals and still stop to jump in a cold river naked. You can be a monster in your pursuit and still build Lego with your daughter while speaking a made-up language only you two understand.
"Wibble flombuckets."
You are not less driven because you laugh.
You are not less ambitious because you stop to taste the fucking strawberries.
You are dangerous because you can do both.

Play Isn't a Distraction. It's a Return.

You were born knowing how to play.
You didn't need to be taught how to laugh.
You didn't need a reason to dance.
You just danced.
Then someone told you to grow up.
To be serious.
To *"act your age."*
They taught you shame.
Taught you guilt.
Taught you that joy was childish.
They were wrong.
Joy isn't childish, it's what makes you whole.
Play is the antidote to rigidity.
And rigid people break.

You want to become the strongest version of yourself?
Reclaim the parts they made you hide.
The curious part.
The silly part.
The part that chuckles in the rain or does stupid dances while cleaning the house.
That's not weakness.
That's freedom.

And freedom terrifies the ones who've built their identity on performance and pain.

Joy Doesn't Diminish Your Fire, It Refuels It.

There's this myth that joy softens you.
That fun makes you lazy.
That if you're laughing, you're not serious enough.
Bullshit.
The happiest fighters I know are also the most deadly.
Because their joy isn't a mask, it's recovery.
Their laughter isn't fake, it's fuel.
They've learned how to fill their own tank, not just keep burning it down.
There's a moment, deep in the grind, when the only thing that'll keep you moving is a small spark of something that reminds you why you started in the first place.
That spark is joy.
Without it, the hustle turns toxic.
Without it, you'll hit your goals and still feel hollow.
Because you weren't building a life - you were just ticking boxes.

Laugh Harder.

The ones who look down on joy?
The ones who roll their eyes at fun?
They're the ones most shackled to the system.
Still performing for invisible applause.
Still chasing a version of success that tastes like ass.
Their seriousness isn't strength - it's fear.
Fear of being seen as soft.
Fear of stopping long enough to feel.
Fear that if they ever took the mask off, there'd be nothing underneath it.
So laugh harder.
Crack the joke.

Sing out of key.
Light the fire pit and howl at the moon if that's what lights your soul.
Because the secret is that the revolution doesn't always look like rage.
Sometimes, it looks like joy.
Big, loud, unashamed joy.
The kind that fills a room and makes people pause.
The kind that says - *"You don't own me.*
I'm still here.
And I'm fucking alive."

Smile Like a Savage.

Smile like someone who's seen the worst and still finds reasons to dance.
Smile like someone who knows joy isn't just allowed - it's essential.
Smile like someone who's rejected the script and written their own rules.
Smile like a savage.
Because joy isn't a soft luxury.
It makes you untouchable.
In a world that wants you dulled down and burnt out, joy is the real act of defiance.
It's the flag you plant in the ground and say - *"This is mine.*
My time.
My peace.
My spark."
So keep your fire raging.
But never forget to laugh while it burns.

Put It On the Table.

Does this 'thought' hit home?
□ Yes   □ Not really

If yes, can you call yourself out and apply it?
□ Yes   □ Still hiding

If yes, what's one move you'll make to prove it's not just words?

....

....

Thought 34
Sanity Is a Moving Target.

You keep trying to pin down sanity like it's a destination. A finish line.
Like one day you'll cross it and finally feel 'normal' again.
Whatever the fuck that means.
The reality nobody's selling in your feed is that sanity isn't static.
It moves.
It bends.
It breaks and reforms.
Some days it walks beside you.
Some days it runs from you.
And the people who survive aren't the ones who stay sane, they're the ones who learn how to function while sanity slips out the back door.
We were sold this lie that mental clarity is some kind of baseline.
That if you eat clean, sleep right, journal and meditate and delete toxic people, you'll feel level.
Bullshit.
Sometimes you can do everything right, and still wake up feeling like your brain's trying to murder you from the inside.
Sometimes the world tips sideways, and you're trapped in a soundtrack that's too loud or too silent.
Sometimes even brushing your teeth feels like negotiating with a hostage-taker.
This doesn't mean you're broken.
It means you're human.
Sanity is a moving target.
You don't aim to hit the bullseye every day - you aim to stay in the game.

Move While the Ground Shifts.

Some people wait for mental stillness before they act.
They think they need clarity to make a decision.
Calm to have the conversation.
Those people get left behind.
Because life doesn't wait for you to feel ready.
Sanity doesn't arrive like a courier package when your schedule
clears. The real ones learn to move through the chaos.
They don't need full access to themselves to take a step forward.
They just need one working limb.
One breath.
One thought that's fire.
That's enough.

You fight with what you've got.
On your best days, you're smooth, sharp, efficient.
On your worst?
You're dragging yourself face-first through gravel.
Doesn't matter.
Still counts.
Still movement.
You learn to adapt.
On the days your mind is fog, you switch to radar.
Feel for the edges.
On the days it's a war zone, you dig trenches.
You build workarounds.
You carry water for yourself like someone you love.
And no, it doesn't always get easier.
That's not the promise here.
The promise is that you get stronger.
Smarter.
More resourceful.
You stop needing ideal conditions.
You stop waiting for the fog to lift before you build.
You learn to build inside it.

Weather Isn't Weakness.

People confuse mental consistency with moral value.
They think if they're off - they're spiralling.
They think if they're not themselves - they're failing.
That it means they're weak.
Unreliable.
Useless.
Wrong.
It just means the weather changed.
Your brain is weather.
Some days it's calm - blue skies and a steady breeze.
Other days it's a fucking hurricane.
Thunder, lightning, howling winds tearing at everything.
You are not the storm.
You are the one walking through it.
And you don't owe anyone sunshine.
You don't need to have perfect posture, clear skin, and a to-do list tattooed on your soul.
You just need to get your arse in the fucking chair and start.
Because that's what mental mastery looks like.
Not perfection.
Not stability.
But resilience.
The ability to work with the chaos, not against it.

When the Mirror Lies.

You will have days that scare you.
Days where you don't recognise your own thoughts.
Where you think things you're not proud of.
Where you stare into the mirror and see a stranger.
Those days aren't warnings - they're invitations.
Invitations to get curious.
To pull the thread.
To ask - "*What part of me is speaking?*
Does it need to be believed, challenged, or simply witnessed?"

Not every thought is an instruction.
Not every feeling is a sign.
Some are echoes from a distant place.
Some are noise cluttering the airwaves.
Some are old scripts your brain forgot to delete.
Let them come.
Let them pass.
You don't need to obey them in order to honour them.
Just notice.
Track the drift.
And if the same darkness keeps circling back, get help.
Not because you're failing, but because you're worth supporting.
Sanity may move, but you don't have to chase it alone.

Performance Is a Prison.

There is a kind of violence in pretending you're fine when you're not.
A kind of psychological self-abandonment.
You split in two -
The version you show the world.
And the one quietly bleeding beneath the surface.
The longer you stay in costume, the harder it gets to breathe.
So stop.
Drop the act.
Not everywhere, not with everyone - just with someone.
Forget performative pain.
This isn't about broadcasting your struggle to rack up hearts and sympathy points.
That's just another mask.
Another performance.
You don't need an audience - you need a witness.
Someone who can hold space while you tell the truth without dressing it up.
Get help.
Real help.
Not just a meme about boundaries or a bath bomb labelled 'self-care.'
I mean the uncomfortable kind.

The kind where you book the session, sit in the chair, and speak the mess out loud.
Therapy.
Counselling.
Coaching.
Whatever gives your thoughts a container and your feelings a name.
Or maybe it's not a professional.
Maybe it's just your person.
That one human who sees past your mask.
Who doesn't cower when you say the hard thing.
Find that person.
Keep them.
Talk to them.
Because silence will rot you if you let it.
You are not meant to carry every weight alone.
And you are not weak for needing to be heard.
Mental health isn't about reaching some final form where you never struggle again.
It's maintenance.
Ongoing.
Gritty.
Sometimes daily.
You clean the wound.
You change the dressing.
You say - *"I'm not okay,"* and let someone answer - *"That's alright, I'm here."*
Healing isn't heroic - it's how you stay human.

Be a Boomerang.

You're allowed to wobble.
You're allowed to contradict yourself -
To believe in your power and feel like a fraud.
To want help and reject it.
To long for connection and isolate.
You are not broken for doing both.
You are human.

Sanity isn't a clean line - it's a heartbeat.
Spiking, dipping, stuttering.
What matters is not that it stays level, but that it keeps going.
So aim less for perfection and more for return.
Return to yourself.
To your values.
To your breath.
Over and over again.
That's the real flex.
Not staying centred like a statue, but finding centre again after you've been knocked sideways.
Every time you come back, you get stronger.
Every time you lose the thread and recover it, your grip improves.
So stop trying to hold onto sanity like it's a fixed thing.
Learn to move with it.
That's how you master the mind.

Put It On the Table.

Does this 'thought' hit home?
☐ Yes   ☐ Not really

If yes, can you call yourself out and apply it?
☐ Yes   ☐ Still hiding

If yes, what's one move you'll make to prove it's not just words?

....

....

Thought 35
The Villain Was Never Real.

The mind's addicted to enemies.
Not because you love the pain, but because it gives you someone to blame.
One face.
One name.
One neat excuse that explains why you're broken, bitter, and stuck.
You weren't just hurt, you were wronged.
And if they're the villain, you get to stay the wounded hero.
But let's kill the fantasy.

The villain was never real.

You didn't find them.
You made them.
Crafted them from shadows and survival instinct, handed them a script, and told them to play the part.
You weren't just the victim - you were the director.
And the story's bullshit.

Memory Lies Like It Loves You.

Memory isn't a photograph.
It's a propaganda reel.
You don't remember the past.
You remember your last version of it.

And every time you revisit that same old story - the betrayal, the rejection, the moment things cracked - you add a little extra colour.
A sharper line here.
A darker tone there.
Over time, the person who hurt you grows fangs.
They morph from human into a full-blown Demogorgon.
Not because they were a monster.
But because your pain needed one to survive.
You don't remember what happened.
You remember how it felt.
And that feeling becomes the whole truth.
But feelings aren't facts.
And distorted memory is a dangerous author.

The Addiction to Blame.

Creating a villain serves a function.
It gives your chaos a shape - a target to aim your blame at.
Convince yourself they fucked you over, and you don't have to face your own mess.
Villains give you a reason to stay angry.
A reason not to try again.
"If they hadn't done that, I'd be miles ahead by now," you say.
But that's a lie you tell yourself to feel safe.
That fantasy is seductive because it absolves you.
Not just from responsibility, but from facing the messy, complicated truth of yourself.
Most people didn't hurt you to hurt you.
They hurt you because they were out of depth, out of tools, or going through their own invisible shit.
You were collateral damage in someone else's storm.
And yeah, that still hurts.
But it's not villainy.
It's dysfunction.
It's misfire.
It's human mess painted in the colours of evil because that made it easier to swallow.

When You're Addicted to the Battle.

Sometimes we don't keep the villain alive because we hate them - we keep them alive because we need them.
Not the person.
The war.
Your whole identity gets braided into the fight.
Without it, who are you?
If you're not the one who was betrayed, rejected, overlooked, what's left?
Who are you without your struggle story?
You get respect for surviving it.
You get comfort for speaking it.
You get a seat at the table because you've bled for it.
So you keep the villain in your back pocket - not as an enemy, but as proof.
Proof that your pain is real.
Proof that your anger is justified.
Proof that you're allowed to stay bitter, unhealed, stuck.
The truth is you don't want revenge.
You want meaning.
You want your suffering to have mattered.
But that meaning will never come from their punishment.
It only comes from your release.
From dropping the weapon.
From realising you were never actually fighting them - you were fighting the part of you that can't imagine life without the war.

Most People Were Just Mirrors.

What if they weren't the villain?
What if they were just the poor bastard reflecting your shit back at you?
Your insecurities.
Your unspoken demands.
The parts of yourself you refuse to face.
People can't read a script you never handed them.

Can't play a role you never had the guts to say out loud.
But when they don't meet your unspoken expectations?
Boom - villain status.

Maybe they didn't betray you.
Maybe they just confused you.
Because you expected them to fix shit they didn't know existed.
You cast them in a play they never auditioned for.
Then you got pissed off when they forgot the lines they were never taught.
Maybe your villains aren't evil - maybe they were just holding the mirror. Cracked, yes.
Flawed, for sure.
But maybe what you saw scared you because it looked too much like you.

The Danger of Narrative Addiction.

We become addicted to our own narratives.
They make sense of the mess.
But once a story sticks, it buries its teeth.
Once you decide someone's a villain, your brain becomes a detective for evidence.
Every cold glance, every sharp word - it all adds to the character profile.
You don't see the full human anymore.
You just see a character in your movie.
And characters don't get nuance.
They get tropes.
That's the danger.
You can't grow if you're still acting in the same script.
Especially one you wrote years ago - under duress, with blood in your mouth and fear in your eyes.

How to Burn the Villain.

So, how do you kill the villain living rent-free in your head?
You don't.
You unwrite them.
You pull back the curtain and realise the role they played was never fixed, it was fabricated.
Not completely false, no.
Pain is real.
Abuse is real.
Betrayal is real.
But villainy?
That's a lens.
And you get to smash that lens whenever you're ready.

Start by naming the story.
Literally say it out loud -
"I made them the villain because it helped me survive.
But I don't need that story anymore."
Then ask the scariest question -
"What will I be without this enemy?"
That's the question most people avoid.
Because once you burn the villain, you burn excuses.
You're no longer reacting.
You're creating.
And that's pure power.

Let Them Go.

This isn't about forgiveness.
You don't need to forgive the version of them that hurt you.
That's not required for your evolution.
But you do need to let go of the version of you who still needs them to be evil.
Because that version of you is stuck in the past.
Frozen in a chapter that ended years ago - and you've got too much ahead to keep rereading the same damn page.

Release doesn't mean reconciliation.
It means taking your power back.
You get to walk away.
Not because they deserve peace, but because you refuse to let them hold your mind hostage any longer.

The End of the Script.

You were never just the hero fighting some external villain.
You were the author, writing every role - the hero, the enemy, the conflict.
It was always you.
And that's the best news you'll ever hear.
Because if you wrote the script, you can rewrite the ending.
No villains.
Just lessons.
Just freedom.
Burn the old script.
And this time, leave no room for monsters.

Put It On the Table.

Does this 'thought' hit home?
☐ Yes   ☐ Not really

If yes, can you call yourself out and apply it?
☐ Yes   ☐ Still hiding

If yes, what's one move you'll make to prove it's not just words?

....

....

Thought 36
Earn the Outcome.

Talent is overrated.
That's not a motivational slogan.
That's a field report.

I'm not talented.
At anything.
Cue sad violin.
And yet, somehow, I've still managed to build things that matter.
Create results.
Cross finish lines.
It's not magic.
It's not luck.
It's effort, stacked day after day, until reality starts paying attention.
That's why I pity people with talent - they've been robbed.
Not of opportunity, but of weight.
They get the thing, but they don't get the wave.
The feeling.
The punch-in-the-gut pride that only comes when you've dragged yourself through the dirt to get it.
For them, the win is clean.
For me, it's tidal.

Same Shoes, Different Story.

Let's play a game.
You want a pair of Jordan 1 Travis Scott sneakers.
The kind that cost more than a month's rent and come wrapped in hype and myth.

Now here are two scenarios.
Scenario 1.
You wake up, shuffle to the front door, and find a box-fresh pair sitting in your postbox.
No name.
No note.
Just a gift from the void.
You shrug.
Try them on.
Snap a pic.
Cool.
Scenario 2.
You save £100 a month for 12 months.
You obsessively trawl the internet for any whiff of a deal.
Finally, you find a seller, but he doesn't post.
He's in Hull.
A city branded 'worst place in the world'.
You drive there.
Your car breaks down 10 miles out.
You start walking.
You get chased by wild dogs.
You arrive, muddy and breathless, only for the seller to change his mind.
But he's got cows that need milking so you make a deal.
Twelve hours later, reeking of bovine sweat and £1,200 lighter, you walk back home.
Sneakers in hand.

Same outcome - box fresh Jordans.
Different reality - one of those stories will live in your bloodstream forever.
The other's a forgettable footnote.
Why?
Because effort changes the result.
It saturates it with meaning.

The Effort Effect.

The outcome doesn't give you the satisfaction.
The earning does.
You can hack, shortcut, inherit, or stumble into a win and still feel
hollow. Because satisfaction doesn't come from the prize - it comes
from knowing what it cost you.
What you gave.
What you became in the process.
That's why I never worry about being talented.
Talent is fast food.
It fills you, but you forget it five minutes later.
Effort is the meal you remember for years.
The one you earned.
The one you bled into.

Your Work Is the Proof.

Every hard-earned win carries fingerprints.
Yours.
Not your potential.
Not your genes.
Not your backstory.
Your sweat.
It proves that you were there.
That you showed up when it didn't make sense to.
That you kept building when no one gave a fuck.
That you gave enough of a shit to get uncomfortable, disciplined,
obsessed.
Because when it's effort, not talent, that gets you across the line - you
own every inch of it.
You don't owe luck a thank-you speech.
You don't owe genetics a nod.
It's yours.
Built from scratch.
And that's where fire comes from - not from ease, but from the pride
of participation.

Stop Worshipping the Gifted.

We glorify the naturally gifted like they've cracked some divine cheat code.
But watch closely.
Talent without effort burns out fast.
The moment things get gritty, unsexy, slow - they bail or plateau.
Because they've never been forced to fight for it.
Effort people are different.
They're forged in the hours no one counts.
The stuff that doesn't get likes, but gets results.
They know that what you lack in talent, you can outwork, outlast, out-grit.
Because fire isn't born.
It's built.

Desire. Discipline. Grit.

You only need three things, and they're available to everyone.
Desire - A reason big enough to drag you through the fog.
Discipline - The system that keeps the flame alive when motivation dies.
Grit - The part of you that doesn't flinch when it's hard, boring, or unclear.

You don't need genius.
You don't need approval.
You don't need a perfect plan.
You just need to stop waiting to be chosen and start choosing yourself.
Again, and again, and again.
Because repetition is how effort carves identity.

Talent Is Not the Point.

Talent might give you a head start - that quick burst of speed when the gun fires, that initial edge that feels like a shortcut.
But talent alone doesn't win the marathon.
Effort builds the whole damn race.
It's the miles you grind out in the rain, the hours you show up when no one's watching, and the relentless pushing past every moment you want to quit.
This isn't about downplaying giftedness or natural ability.
It's about refusing to be paralysed by its absence.
You are not stuck.
You're just not pushing hard enough, long enough, or consistently enough.
Not because you can't, but because you haven't yet made that choice.
You think the universe is holding out on you?
Holding back opportunities, waiting for you to "*deserve*" success?
It's not.
The universe doesn't play favourites - it simply waits for you to get serious.
To build anyway.
To earn anyway.
To do the fucking work.

The Only Satisfaction That Lasts.

The satisfaction that lasts the longest is the one that came hardest.
It's the one that bruised you.
That tested your resolve.
That took too long, cost too much, and almost made you quit.
That's the one that builds the legend inside you.
Because what you had to work for becomes part of your wiring.
It changes the way you walk.
It changes what you tolerate.
It changes what you expect from yourself.
That's not just achievement - that's internal transformation.

Earn It Because You Can.

You don't need to be special.
You don't need to be the best.
You just need to be relentless.
Because there's nothing sweeter than standing at the end of a long,
ugly road, holding the thing you swore you'd get, knowing that no one
gave it to you.
Knowing it wasn't talent.
It wasn't luck.
It was you.
Every inch of it.
Earned.
And that satisfaction?
That wave?
That's the whole fucking point.

Put It On the Table.

Does this 'thought' hit home?
☐ Yes   ☐ Not really

If yes, can you call yourself out and apply it?
☐ Yes   ☐ Still hiding

If yes, what's one move you'll make to prove it's not just words?

....

....

Thought 37
Not All Silence Is Peace.

Silence wears disguises.
Sometimes it's strength.
Sometimes it's decay.
Sometimes it's the calm before a breakthrough.
Sometimes it's the sound of someone slowly disappearing from themselves.
Stillness can deceive - not every silence is peaceful.

Some People Go Quiet Because They've Given Up.

Let's stop romanticising stillness.
Some people go quiet not because they're grounded, but because they've tapped out.
They've stopped showing up.
Not because they've found 'balance' or 'alignment', but because they're tired of failing.
Tired of wanting.
Tired of trying.
Tired of hearing their own excuses echo back.
And so they shrink.
They start skipping the workout.
Skipping the calls.
Skipping the life they once swore they were building.
They ghost their own goals like they were just a phase.
Then they wrap it up with soft language.
"It's not that deep."
"I'm just taking it slow right now."
"I'm chilling."

Wrong.
They're not chilling.
They're folding.
They've muted the hunger, not because they don't want it, but because they're scared they can't have it.
And that kind of silence?
That's not calm.
That's corrosion.
The kind that doesn't scream, erupt or explode - it just leaks.
Until one day, there's nothing left to lose because there's nothing left of you.

And Then There's the Other Kind.

Not all silence is surrender.
There's another kind of quiet that should scare the fuck out of people.
The kind that simmers.
The kind that hums.
The kind that doesn't ask for attention because it's busy becoming the answer.
That silence?
That's someone in the lab.
Someone dialled in.
Tuned out.
Focused so hard they forgot the world existed.
They're not ignoring you, they've just locked in on something louder than validation.
They've gone dark so they can get brighter.
They're quiet because they're building something worth the noise.
They don't need to prove anything.
They'll let the result do the talking.

The Outside Doesn't Always Match the Inside.

Here's where people get lost - they think energy equals volume.

They think visibility equals progress.
They think noise equals momentum.
Lies.
Some of the loudest voices are empty echoes.
All post, no power.
All bark, no plan.
All dopamine, no direction.
And some of the quietest?
Meanwhile, some of the quietest souls are sitting on volcanoes -
smouldering with ideas, fuelled by discipline, brimming with energy.
They're waiting.
Building.
Layering.
Just because someone's not shouting doesn't mean they're not rising.
Just because someone's not broadcasting doesn't mean they're not
growing.
So stop measuring heat by how much smoke you see.
Start watching habits.
Start watching patterns.
Start watching what happens over time, not what's trending right now.
Because real moves don't beg for claps.
They just land.

You've Got to Check Your Own Silence Too.

This isn't just about other people.
Turn the mirror around.
Your silence, what's it made of?
Is it power or pause?
Is it vision or avoidance?
Is it strategy or straight-up surrender?
Be honest.
Some people call it peace because it sounds better than stuck.
Some call it solitude because numb feels too raw.
Some call it reflection because hiding feels too shameful.

There's a thin line between stillness and stagnation.
And the longer you pretend not to notice which side you're on, the deeper it digs in.
Ask yourself - is your quiet building something?
Or is it just a padded room you've convinced yourself is a temple?

Peace Has a Pulse.

Peace isn't passive.
It breathes.
It moves.
It beats.
Peace is not lying flat, waiting for the world to sort itself out.
It's not unplugging from your life and calling it detachment.
It's not zoning out and branding it alignment.
Peace is sharp.
Peace is clean.
Peace has edges.
It comes after confrontation, not in place of it.
It's what rises after you've looked yourself in the face, sorted your shit, and decided who's driving next.
Real peace doesn't look like a monk floating above the chaos.
It looks like someone who walked through the fire, learned its temperature, and came back with direction.
Peace is built.
Earned.
Lived.
It's not what you find at the end of a yoga class.
It's what you build when you stop lying to yourself.

Know the Difference.

You might be quiet right now.
Fine.
But what's your silence saying?

Does it signal progress or protection?
Does it whisper growth or guilt?
Does it feel like a sanctuary or a cell?
Not all silence is peace.
Some people go quiet because they've stopped believing in themselves.
Others go quiet because they're done performing and ready to create.
Figure out which one you are.
And if you're on the wrong side of that line?
Get up.
Wake the fuck up.
Reignite the signal.
Make noise with your work.
Make noise with your effort.
Let your silence carry weight, not dust.
Because peace isn't found in the dark.
It's made when you finally step back into the light and own your next move like it's the only thing that matters.

Put It On the Table.

Does this 'thought' hit home?
☐ Yes   ☐ Not really

If yes, can you call yourself out and apply it?
☐ Yes   ☐ Still hiding

If yes, what's one move you'll make to prove it's not just words?

....

....

Part 5

FULL FUCKING OWNERSHIP

Thought 38
Only Dead Fish Go With the Flow.

When was the last time you truly asked yourself why?
Why are you in that job?
Why are you chasing that title?
Why do you dress like that, speak like that, post like that?
Most of the time, the answer isn't *"because I want to."*
It's *"because I thought I should."*
'Should' is the quiet killer.
It's where your edge gets sanded down.
Where you swap freedom for approval.
And then one day, you realise you've built a life to impress people you don't even like.
And the worst part?
You don't even know who to blame.
Because it wasn't one big decision.
It was a thousand tiny agreements.
A thousand silent nods to things that didn't feel right, but felt expected.
That's how you end up numb.
Tamed.
Beige.

Beige Living and the Lie of the Path.

We're taught to play small.
Fit in.
Be neat.

Keep your head down.
Go to school.
Get the job.
Buy the house.
Marry someone acceptable.
Raise two kids with no questions.
Retire quietly.
That's the flow.
That's the template.
And the people following it?
Dead fish.
No spark.
No challenge.
Just driftwood in dress shirts.
But the second you turn and swim the other way?
You're - *"Reckless."*
"Selfish."
"Delusional."

Perfect.

It means you've stopped pretending.
You've clocked the con.
Because that tidy little path they sold you?
The one paved with promises and promotions?
It's fiction.
A fucking fairy tale for the obedient.
There's no master rulebook.
No divine checklist.
No scoreboard tracking your good behaviour.
The real win?
It's power.
Not over others - over yourself.
The kind that comes when you stop putting on a show.
When you tear up the script and live without a fucking filter.
When you get loud.
Get raw.

Get real.
And finally build a life that answers to no one but you.

Your Weird Is the Whole Point.

You're not a universal adapter.
You were never made to please the masses.
You're weird.
Niche.
The moment you stop twisting to be liked?
Everything clicks.
You shed the weight.
Your people find you.
You start breathing properly.
You stop asking permission.
You become the permission.
And that weirdness you've been hiding?
That thing that makes you feel - *"too much,"* *"too intense,"* *"too out there"*?
That's your power.

History doesn't belong to the well-behaved - it belongs to the ones who stood out and refused to blend.
So let them stare.
Let them whisper.
Let them get uncomfortable.
You weren't made to blend.

Outlaws Over Echoes.

The world doesn't need more echoes.
It doesn't need another feed full of influencers repeating borrowed dreams.
It needs outlaws.
People who move like they mean it.
Who build strange, messy, defiant lives.

The ones who scare people a little.
Who refuse to be muted.
Be that.
Not digestible.
Not predictable.
Not a replica of anyone else.
Be the one they can't box in.
Be the one they remember when the dust settles.
Be the outlaw.
Be powerful.

Kill the Apology.

Stop apologising for wanting more.
More fire.
More space.
More you.
You're not "*too much.*"
You're just too alive for the half-life you've been offered.
Every time you shrink to soothe someone else's discomfort, a piece of you starves.
Start feeding yourself instead.
Take up room.
Say what you mean.
Make the damn noise.
You're not here to be small and agreeable.
You're here to take up your full fucking shape.
Kill the apology before it kills your spark.

Break the Inheritance.

Not everything you were handed is worth keeping.
The rules.
The roles.
The recycled fears passed down like old furniture.
You can love your people and still torch their blueprint.

You can respect your roots and still refuse to live by them.
Legacy isn't built through compliance - it's forged in courage.
Be the one who stops the cycle.
Be the one who redraws the map.
You are not obligated to carry the weight of ghosts.
Be the break.

Build Without Blueprints.

We're obsessed with having a plan.
Ten-year goals.
Vision boards.
Step-by-step life timelines.
We treat life like it's a school project - something to be mapped, ticked off, and graded.
But life isn't tidy.
It's wild.
Chaotic.
Alive.
And if you're always waiting for the perfect plan?
You'll never fucking move.
You'll sit on your best ideas until they wither.
You'll analyse every fork in the road until it disappears under your feet.
You'll mistake perfectionism for progress and stall your own becoming.
Clarity doesn't come from thinking.
It comes from doing.
Not theorising.
Not waiting for a sign from the universe.
You learn what works by starting.
You learn who you are by choosing.
You find your rhythm by walking headfirst into the unknown.

You don't need to know how it ends.
You just need to begin.
And yes, it will be messy.
You'll change your mind.

You'll take wrong turns.
You'll build things that fall apart.
But that's the point.
That's the process.
Stop waiting to feel ready.
Start before the fear wears off.
Start before you have permission.

Blueprints are for replicas.
You're not here to repeat someone else's architecture - you're here to invent.
Build your life the way artists build paintings -
Layer by layer.
Mistake by mistake.
Stroke by stroke.
Until one day, it stops looking like a plan and starts looking like something breathtaking.
Not because it's perfect.
But because it's yours.

Swim the Other Way.

If safety's your goal, go with the flow.
The current will carry you to the same quiet shore as everyone else - predictable, beige, unbothered.
You won't drown.
But you won't live either.
But if you want a life with teeth?
Against the pull.
Against the script.
Against every easy "yes" that keeps you small.
Kick until your legs burn.
Claw until your hands are raw.
Break rank even when every voice around you says - "Stay in line."
Make people uncomfortable.
Make systems glitch.
Make the algorithm choke on your unpredictability.

Normal doesn't need another recruit.
It's already overstaffed.
You weren't born to be palatable.
You weren't born to colour inside the lines.
You were made to disrupt.
To build.
To burn.
Be the one that swims until the river bends to you.

And if people don't get it?
Let them drift.
Only dead fish go with the flow.

Put It On the Table.

Does this 'thought' hit home?
☐ Yes ☐ Not really

If yes, can you call yourself out and apply it?
☐ Yes ☐ Still hiding

If yes, what's one move you'll make to prove it's not just words?

....

....

Thought 39

You Don't Need to Be Happy, You Need to Be Whole.

You don't need to be happy.
Not all the time.
Not even most of the time.
This modern obsession with happiness is doing more damage than good.
We treat happiness like a destination, like something we're meant to arrive at and then just stay there.
Forever smiling, drinking green juice, and radiating positivity like a human fucking lighthouse.
Reality check.
That's not life.
That's a Netflix ad.
And here's the dangerous part - chasing it can make you more miserable than whatever you were trying to escape in the first place.

The Lie of Constant Happiness.

You're not broken because you feel like shit.
You're not failing because you're tired, lost, angry, anxious, or just numb.
You're human.
The real problem is that we've been sold this toxic idea that unless we're happy, we're doing life wrong.

So we start chasing it.
New job.
New body.
New partner.
New car.
New dopamine hit.
And when that doesn't work, we double down.
Smile more.
Fake it.
Post it.
Polish it.
Pretend.
And every time that doesn't fix the unhappiness, we think something must be wrong with us.
Spoiler alert - nothing's wrong with you.
You're just playing by a set of rules that are rigged to keep you chasing.

Look around...
Entire industries are built on your discontent.
Marketing, self-help, beauty, wellness - they all whisper the same thing - "*You're not enough yet.*
But buy this, do this, become this - and maybe you will be."
It's a con.
One designed to keep you on the treadmill, panting for joy that's always two steps out of reach.
We don't need more tips on how to smile our way through pain.
We need permission to stop pretending.

You're a Full Fucking Spectrum.

You weren't designed to feel one emotion forever.
You're a walking contradiction.
Light and dark, calm and chaos, joy and grief, love and fury.
That's not a glitch.
That's the whole design.
Feeling sad?

That's data.
Feeling rage?
That's truth.
Feeling hollow?
That's a sign.
Don't ignore it.
Don't numb it.
Don't hashtag positivity over it.
Feel the thing.
Process it.
Own it.
Then move.

Real strength is not pretending everything's fine.
It's learning how to sit in the fire without losing yourself in it.
Emotions aren't the enemy, they're messages.
When you feel despair, it may be because something needs to change.
When you feel joy, that's a breadcrumb pointing you toward what matters.
The moment you start treating your emotions like a compass instead of a curse, you take your power back.
We've been trained to identify ourselves with our feelings.
"I'm anxious."
"I'm broken."
But you're not.
You're experiencing anxiety.
You're feeling overwhelmed.
There's a difference.
A storm passing through isn't the sky.
You're not your weather - you're the whole atmosphere.

The Hustle for Happiness is Making You Miserable.

We grind.
We perform.

We compare.
We optimise.
All in the name of being happy.
But half the time, what we really want is peace.
What we need is wholeness.
To be seen, accepted, understood - not by the crowd, but by ourselves.
You're not here to be 'good vibes only'.
You're here to be fucking real.
And that means honouring all of it.
The joy.
The trauma.
The wild ideas.
The deep insecurities.
The days where you feel bulletproof, and the days where you can't get out of bed.
That's what it means to be whole.
To be fully you, not just the parts that are easy to post.
The world screams at us to constantly improve.
Upgrade.
Reinvent.
There's an entire culture obsessed with turning you into a project -
Biohack your brain.
Wake up at 5am.
Journal.
Meditate.
Take cold showers.
None of these things are bad.
But if you're doing them because you think you need to fix yourself to be lovable, you're missing the fucking point.
Self-improvement without self-acceptance is just self-rejection dressed up in a nicer outfit.
The endless pursuit of 'better' can quietly convince you you're never enough as you are.
And that's where the burnout creeps in.
Not from doing too much, but from never feeling like you're allowed to just be.

Being Whole > Being Happy.

Look, happiness is great.
When it's real, it's golden.
But wholeness?
Wholeness is bulletproof.
Happiness is conditional.
It asks *"are things going well?*
Are you winning?"
Wholeness doesn't care if the house is on fire.
It says, *"I know who I am inside the ashes."*
Wholeness is knowing that even when you feel weak, you're still worthy.
Even when you feel broken, you're still building.
Even when the voice in your head is loud, you're still here.
Still fighting.
And that?
That's fucking beautiful.

You won't always feel good.
Some mornings will come with grief in your bones.
Some nights will swallow you whole.
But if you've done the work of becoming whole, those moments don't define you.
They shape you.
You don't chase wholeness. You build it. Brick by brutal brick.
Through honesty.
Through facing your shit.
Through forgiving the past.
Through owning the present.

Wholeness Over Hype.

So no, you don't need to be happy all the time.
You don't need to force a smile when your soul's screaming.
You don't need to be a walking Instagram quote.
You need to be whole.

Fully human.
Fully flawed.
Fully present.
Let go of this pressure to feel good 24/7.
Let go of the shame when you don't.
Let go of the lie that pain makes you weak.
And next time someone asks how you're doing, don't feel the need to say, *"I'm good"* just to make them comfortable.
If you're struggling, say it.
Let them hear it.
Let them sit with it.
If you're soaring, own it.
Don't apologise for your brightness.
If you're somewhere in the middle, welcome to the club.
There's a richness there that no highlight reel can show.
Stop chasing highs.
Stop measuring yourself by smiles, likes, or applause.
Start building the ground beneath your feet.
Strength isn't in the peaks.
It's in the layers of your days - the quiet work, the decisions you make when no one's watching, the consistency that shows up even when you don't feel like it.
Stop chasing the high and start building the ground beneath you.
The real flex?
Feeling everything without needing to fix everything.
You don't need to be happy.
You just need to be real.
And real is enough.

Put It On the Table.

Does this 'thought' hit home?
□ Yes   □ Not really

If yes, can you call yourself out and apply it?
□ Yes   □ Still hiding

If yes, what's one move you'll make to prove it's not just words?

....

....

Thought 40
Stop Looking for the Map.

Everyone's looking for the blueprint.
The steps.
The guide.
The proven path.
"What's the secret to success?"
"How did they do it?"
"What's the trick?"
Here's the truth…
There is no trick.
There's no fucking map.
You're the map.

And the longer you wait for someone else to show you how to get to where you want to be, the longer you'll stay exactly where you are.
Stuck in the same old place.
Holding out hope that someone will give you permission to start your life.

The World Loves a Checklist.

Life comes pre-loaded with a checklist.
Do this.
Don't do that.
Follow these rules.
Take these steps.
Study this.
Get that job.
Marry that type of person.

Buy a house.
Save X amount.
Retire at 65.
Clap politely at your funeral.
It's all scripted.
Predictable.
Sanitised.
Everything's built to condition us to follow someone else's version of what a 'good life' looks like.
So when we hit the real world and realise there's no clear path?
We freeze.
"Where's the structure?"
"What am I supposed to do now?"
"Who's going to tell me how to do this?"
No one.
Because no one knows the way.
You're meant to create it.
And that truth is terrifying.
We've been spoon-fed certainty.
So when we're finally handed a blank page, we panic.
We try to Google our way to destiny.
We wait for signs, wait for clarity, wait for the stars to align.
As if someone, somewhere, is going to deliver a personalised life plan like a fucking Amazon package.
They won't.
No one's coming.
And that's good news.

My Grandfather Didn't Find a Map.

This thought was inspired by my grandfather.
An orphan.
Troubled beginnings.
No silver spoon, no safety net.
He lived on a park bench.
Worked as a bouncer on the door of a brothel.

Was deported from Calais.
Scraped together a living selling junk he dug out of a dump.
He didn't follow anyone's rules.
He didn't wait for a breakthrough.
He didn't ask for directions.
He made his own luck.
Drew his own line.
And backed himself.
Every.
Single.
Day.
By the time he died, he was a wealthy man.
Happily married.
Three kids.
Three grandkids who loved and respected the ground he walked on.
He didn't have a map.
He had balls, resilience, grit, and heart.
And that was enough.
He showed me something no curriculum ever did.
That if you want a life that matters, you build it from scratch.
With blood, sweat, and stubborn hope.

Waiting for the Map Is Just Fear in Disguise.

You say you're not ready.
You're waiting for the perfect time.
The right opportunity.
The 'sign'.
But that's not strategy.
That's fear disguised as control.
You want a guarantee.
You want certainty.
You want someone to point and say - "Go that way, success is over there."
It doesn't work like that.
You want clarity?

Create it.
You want purpose?
Pick something.
Build something.
Bleed for something.
You want progress?
Start moving, even if you don't know where it'll end up.
Waiting is comfortable.
It's clean.
Safe.
Sterile.
You get to dream big without risking a fall.
But movement?
Movement costs you - it'll demand your doubt, your sleep, your ego.
But that's the price of momentum.
You don't get to know how it ends before you begin.
That's not courage, that's control.
And life doesn't work on your terms.

Every Wrong Turn Teaches You Something.

There is no clean route.
No shortcut.
No smooth, paved road.
You'll fuck up.
You'll zig when you should've zagged.
You'll lose time, lose people, maybe even lose yourself for a bit.
But that's not failure.
That's cartography.
The map is being drawn with every mistake.
Every scar on your journey becomes a marker.
Every loss?
Coordinates.
Every lesson?
A landmark.
That's how you map your way forward.

The detours, the heartbreaks, the wreckage - they become your curriculum.
And they teach you more than any TED Talk ever will.
You're not supposed to get it right on the first try.
You're supposed to get in the ring, get knocked around, then get back up and say - *"Alright, not that way.*
Let's try something else."
That's how you figure out where you're going.
By learning, not knowing.

Everyone You Admire Started With Nothing But a Blank Page.

Those people you respect?
They didn't follow a script.
They weren't handed a plan.
They just started walking.
Blind.
Broke.
Bold.
Figuring it out as they went.
Taking risks.
Taking hits.
Taking ownership.
Sometimes falling flat on their faces.
Sometimes doubting themselves.
And that's what you need to do.
No more waiting.
No more researching the 'right way'.
No more daydreaming about what you could be if someone just showed you how.
Stop romanticising the people who've made it and start doing what they did.
They didn't wait for a map.
They just fucking started.
You don't see the flailing, the fear, the 3 a.m. tears.
You see the results.
The shine.

The destination.
But every journey started messy.
The only difference between them and you?
They stopped waiting.
They picked up the pen.
They started drawing the damn map.

Be the Cartographer.

You don't need anyone's permission.
You don't need someone else's structure.
You don't need a clear path.
You need to move.
You need to commit.
You need to stop waiting and start building.
Even when the floor feels shaky.
Even when the light flickers.
Even when everyone tells you it's impossible.
And yeah, it'll be messy.
You'll doubt yourself.
People will question you.
You'll question yourself more.
You'll ask if it's worth it.
You'll curse your own ambition.
But one day, someone will look at the life you've created and say -
"How the hell did you get there?"
And you'll say - *"I stopped looking for the map.*
And I made one."
Maybe it's not perfect.
Maybe it's jagged, chaotic, and full of wrong turns.
But it's yours.
Built with your hands, your hurt, your hope.
That matters more than anything polished you could've copied.
Because the people who make their own maps become guides for others.
Not because they knew the way.
But because they walked it anyway.

So here's to those who blaze without a torch.
To those who march without a manual.
To those who start with nothing and still choose to begin.
I dedicate this thought to the OG Hoppy - Peter Hopkinson,
who lived by the motto -
"*Save time, see it my way.*"

Put It On the Table.

Does this 'thought' hit home?
☐ Yes   ☐ Not really

If yes, can you call yourself out and apply it?
☐ Yes   ☐ Still hiding

If yes, what's one move you'll make to prove it's not just words?

....

....

Thought 41
Burn the Boats.

There's a story, maybe you've heard it.
A military leader lands on enemy shores.
Outnumbered.
Outgunned.
Zero room for error.
And what's the first thing he orders?

"Burn the boats!"

That's it.
No escape.
No retreat.
No safety net.
Just one option -
Win or die trying.
And guess what?
They won.
Not because they were the strongest.
Not because they had the best plan or the best gear.
Not because luck fell in their lap or because someone held their hand.
But because they had no way back.
The only direction was forward.
The only option was all in.
That story isn't about war.
It's about life.
It's about you.
Because right now, there's something you want, something you're
chasing.
But if you're still clinging to the boats, you're not really chasing it.

You're just entertaining the idea of it.
You're flirting with it from the safety of the shoreline.

Comfort Is a Liar.

Most people say they want to change.
They talk a good game.
"*I want to level up.*"
"*I want more out of life.*"
"*I'm ready to do what it takes.*"
But when it comes time to commit, really commit -
They hedge.
They keep one foot in the past.
They leave the back door cracked open.
They play both sides.
"*If this doesn't work, I'll just fall back on xyz*"
"*I'll give it a shot, but I'm not going all in.*"
"*Let's see how it goes.*"
That isn't ambition.
That's comfort whispering in your ear - "*Stay safe, stay small.*"
And you'll listen, because comfort makes a compelling argument.
Gather more information.
Perfect the plan.
Wait for everyone's approval.
But comfort's a dirty liar.
It wants you calm, quiet, predictable.
Comfort kills potential more efficiently than failure ever could.
Because failure teaches while comfort sedates.
And you can't grow while you're numbing.

Burning the Boats Means You Go All In.

You want to get clean?
Burn the boats.
You want to leave the job you hate and build something that matters?

Burn the boats.
You want to be the fittest, sharpest, most dangerous version of yourself?
Burn.
The.
Fucking.
Boats.
It means no more fallback.
No more - "*I'll try.*"
It means committing with blood in your teeth.
You burn the comfort.
You burn the excuses.
You burn the illusion that you can do something extraordinary with a backup plan waiting in the wings.
You're either in or you're out.
There is no middle ground.
The middle ground is where dreams go to rot.

Most People Never Go All In.

Most people flirt with commitment.
They dabble.
They dip a toe, then run when the water's cold.
They talk big, but move small.
They make vision boards instead of bleeding for it.
They manifest instead of acting.
They wait for the 'right time' - as if time gives a shit.
They stay in the relationship that's dead.
They keep the job that's killing their soul.
They cling to a routine that numbs instead of ignites.
Why?
Because going all in is brutal.
It's a declaration of war against mediocrity.
And most people don't want a war, they want comfort with a side of achievement.
But the ones who win?
The ones who actually change their lives?

They're the ones who say -
"*I'm done waiting.*"
"*I'm not asking for permission.*"
"*I'm not here to play it safe.*"
"*I'm here to fucking conquer.*"
They go in without a net.
Without a second plan.
Without the bullshit story that failure would be too hard to survive.
They bet it all on themselves.
And yeah, it's terrifying.
That's the point.

Going All In Hurts.

Burning the boats is not glamorous.
It's not a cinematic moment with motivational music.
It's gritty.
It's bloody.
It's lonely as fuck.
It means you can't quit when it gets hard.
It means you show up even when you're exhausted, unsure, and embarrassed.
It means you fall, get up, and fall again, and there's no soft landing.
It's the day you delete the contact you shouldn't keep.
It's the moment you walk away from comfort without a plan B.
It's the night you cry on the floor and still decide to go again in the morning.
Burning the boats strips you of your options.
And in that brutal clarity, you find your power.
Because without escape, your only choice is evolution.
You adapt.
You push.
You get resourceful.
You figure it the fuck out.
You don't just grow - you become a weapon.
When you back yourself into a corner and fight like hell, you discover parts of you that comfort could never awaken.

Discipline.
Focus.
Ferocity.
It's not clean.
It's not pretty.
But it's real.
And real is what builds things that last.

Let's Fucking Go.

Burning the boats isn't loud.
It's not a war cry or a chest beat.
It's a private reckoning.
No cameras.
No crowd.
No playlist swelling in the background.
Just you, facing the choice you've dodged a hundred times.
You stare down the old life - the habits, the stories, the back doors you've kept open - and you say - "No more."
Not with drama.
With certainty.
You don't need another motivational hit.
You don't need someone to hype you up or map out the perfect plan.
You need to decide.
No more maybe.
No more waiting for signs.
No more dipping a toe in and calling it commitment.
This is about resolve.
It's about drawing the line, and then walking past it without looking back.

You won't feel ready.
You won't feel brave.
But you'll move anyway.
Because something inside you knows...
It's time.
The old life has served its sentence.

The boats have done their job.
Now they burn.
And as the smoke rises behind you, there's only one thing left to do -
Start walking.

Put It On the Table.

Does this 'thought' hit home?
☐ Yes   ☐ Not really

If yes, can you call yourself out and apply it?
☐ Yes   ☐ Still hiding

If yes, what's one move you'll make to prove it's not just words?

....

....

Thought 42
Built in the Dark.

Everyone wants the light.
The recognition.
The reward.
The proof.
The applause that says - *"You made it."*
But what they forget is that everything worth anything is built in the dark.
Not in front of a crowd.
Not under spotlights.
Not with a standing ovation or a flood of likes.
It's built early.
Late.
Quietly.
Repetitively.
When your head's heavy, your heart's unsure, and your motivation's on life support - but you still show up.
Because the grind that no one sees is the one that shapes you.
That's the one that saves you.

Your Reputation Is Built in Public, Your Identity Is Built in Private.

Anyone can talk.
Anyone can post quotes and preach discipline when the mood is right.
Anyone can be driven when eyes are on them.
But real ones are built in silence.
They're built in the 5 a.m. wake-up, when the bed feels like a trap.
They're built in the cold garage gym where there's no music, no mirror, no acting.

They're built in the kitchen at night, meal prepping when takeout would be easier.
They're built at the desk, in the notebook, on the run, in the reps - when quitting would go unnoticed, and still, you don't.
You become dangerous when you realise the world doesn't need to see your effort for it to matter.
You don't need a witness.
You just need to keep swinging.
Because when you build in the dark, you stop relying on praise to stay consistent.
You stop being driven by validation.
You start being driven by vision.
By purpose.
By obsession.
That's what makes you bulletproof.

You Learn to Love the Boring.

Most people don't quit because it's hard.
They quit because it's boring.
Discipline is mundane.
Progress is repetitive.
Improvement is painfully slow.
You want to talk about growth?
It looks like writing one more paragraph when you'd rather scroll.
Lifting one more rep when no one's counting.
Saying no to the easy out.
Saying yes to the unglamorous task.
Waking up early.
Again.
And again.
And again.
There's no recognition.
There's no viral moment.
There's just you, doing the thing, again.
And if you can stomach the boredom?
You'll outperform 90% of people who only move when it's exciting.

You'll separate from the crowd not with drama, but with discipline.
Everyone wants to be elite until they realise that elite really means mastering monotony.
Finding your edge in repetition.
Becoming lethal in the lulls.

I Run in the Rain.

I've got this thing.
I love running in the pissing rain.
Not a soft drizzle - I mean sideways, skin-stinging, sock-drenching, zero-visibility kind of rain.
And while I'm out there - legs aching, breath burning, shoes soaked - I always picture the same scene.
Everyone else inside.
Sofa life.
Hot chocolate.
Blanket.
Netflix humming.
Safe.
Comfortable.
Sedated.
And I smile.
Not because I think I'm better.
But because I know I'm choosing what most won't.
I'm choosing the discomfort.
I'm choosing the dark.
Because out there, soaked and unseen, is where I'm sharpening the blade.
There's no crowd.
No endorphin hit from being noticed.
There's just effort.
There's just forward motion.
The rain doesn't care about your excuses.
It punishes the weak and challenges the committed.
It reminds you that comfort is a trap and consistency is a weapon.

And that's why I keep running.
Because the reps you do when no one's watching are the ones that make you a savage when they finally do.

Why the Dark Matters.

The dark gets a bad rap.
People think it's where you get lost.
Where you wander.
Where you suffer.
Where failure festers and fear breeds.
But the dark is where you get built.
It's where distraction dies.
It's where ego burns.
It's where clarity lives.
Because when there's no audience, there's no act.
Just truth.
You want to meet the real you?
Turn off the lights.
Silence the crowd.
See what's left when the hype fades.
If you can sit in that?
And still move?
Still grow?
You've got something real.
Most people want results, not refinement.
But if you want to become unshakable you don't just build skill - you build self.

When the Lights Come On, You'll Be Ready.

Let everyone else chase visibility.
You chase capacity.
Because when the moment arrives and opportunity finally knocks - you won't blink.

You won't choke.
You won't scramble to prepare.
You'll step up like you've been there before.
Because you have.
In the mornings no one saw.
In the nights no one praised.
In the grind no one clapped for.
In the silence, you learned.
In the solitude, you sharpened.

You didn't wait for the spotlight.
You became the type of person who could handle it.
That's the whole point.
Not to impress people.
But to be ready when it matters.
Because they can take away the crowd, cut the mic, shut the lights.
But if you've been built in the dark?
You'll still rise.

Build Quiet. Strike Loud.

There's something terrifying about a person who builds in silence.
They don't announce their hustle.
They don't explain their moves.
They don't beg for attention.
They just appear - evolved.
Suddenly sharper.
Suddenly faster.
Suddenly undeniable.
And the world says - *"Where the fuck did that come from?"*
The dark mate - that's where.
So if you're grinding right now and no one's noticing?
Stay there.
Stay hidden.
Stay focused.

Let them forget you.
Let them doubt you.
Let them think you've slowed down.
Then step out.
No warning.
No speech.
Just results so loud they shake the fucking ground.
Because when you build in the dark, you don't just surprise the world
-
You redefine it.

Put It On the Table.

Does this 'thought' hit home?
☐ Yes   ☐ Not really

If yes, can you call yourself out and apply it?
☐ Yes   ☐ Still hiding

If yes, what's one move you'll make to prove it's not just words?

....

....

Thought 43

Superpowers You Didn't Know You Had.

Some powers don't look like powers.
They don't come with capes.
They don't come with applause.
They don't get posted with a motivational quote and a perfect sunrise.
They come wrapped in pain.
In pressure.
In past versions of yourself you'd rather forget.
But once you recognise them for what they are, you realise you've been holding nuclear energy this whole time - you just didn't know how to use it.
Here are three superpowers most people never talk about.
The kind forged in fire.
The kind you only earn by surviving shit no one else sees.

1. Financial Struggle.

Being broke is a pressure cooker.
Not just on your wallet - on your sense of worth, your identity, your ability to breathe without checking the overdraft.
You learn to live with your shoulders tight, scanning every decision like it's a security risk.
Every choice feels amplified, every step costly.
But inside that chaos is a gift most people never get.
Relentless resourcefulness.
Because when you're skint, you don't wait for the perfect plan.
You don't fantasise.
You fucking move.

You get creative.
Strategic.
Brutally efficient.
You sharpen instincts that people with cushioned lives never get to access.
You learn how to flip £20 into three meals and a new side hustle.
You learn how to stretch energy when you're running on caffeine and fumes.
You learn how to make a way, because no one's coming to make it for you.
That kind of urgency burns through excuses.
That kind of pressure turns hesitation into momentum.
That kind of scarcity teaches you speed, strategy, and stamina.
And once you've survived like that?
Once you've built momentum with nothing but scraps and stubbornness?
Money stops being the master.
You stop chasing pounds for validation.
You start building value because you are the asset.
You become dangerous not because you're rich, but because you know that even if they took it all away, you'd find a way again.
You learn to fight with your hands tied - and that fight becomes freedom.

2. Rivalry.

Sibling rivalry is a weird beast.
It's not about hate.
It's not even about competition in the usual sense.
It's about pace.
If you've got siblings, you know the feeling.
They get a promotion, and something in your gut tightens.
They post a photo from some slick new holiday, and your brain goes straight to your own passport, your own progress.
They win, you feel it.
They level up, and you start scanning the map for your next move.

Not because you want them to lose.
Not because you're bitter.
But because something deep in you refuses to fall behind.
There's a primal spark that comes from growing up side by side with someone who's constantly pushing you just by existing.
You measure yourself in shadows and milestones.
And when that rivalry's healthy it's rocket fuel.
You move quicker.
You recover faster.
It teaches you not to rest on your wins.
Not to coast.
Rivalry, when it's clean, breeds quiet accountability.
It creates internal standards.
It sharpens your eye for bullshit, especially your own.
And even if you love them, even if you're proud as hell of them - you still want your own name in the story.
You want your own wins.
Your own version of glory.
And that's okay.
That edge is not toxic.
It's ancestral.
It's what keeps the bloodline from fading into mediocrity.
What turns siblings into catalysts?
Mirrors and benchmarks.
The game isn't about beating them.
It's about becoming the kind of person they'd have to chase, too.

3. Grief.

If you've ever grieved, really grieved, you know what I mean.
You come back different.
Not softer.
Not stronger.
Just different.
There's a clarity that follows loss.
Not the kind that whispers.
The kind that punches.

You see life through a new lens.
The noise quiets.
The fake stuff melts.
The small talk dies.
When you've been cracked open by loss, when you've stood at the edge of the abyss and looked into it, you stop getting rattled by the trivial.
Someone cuts you off in traffic?
Whatever.
Your project deadline gets moved?
Not worth the adrenaline.
Some idiot talks behind your back?
You don't even flinch.
Because you've already faced the thing most people dread - the brutal truth that everything can be ripped from you.
That kind of pain rewires you.
It teaches you what's real.
What's worth your energy.
What's just background noise trying to pass for importance.
You learn not to waste time.
Not because you're scared but because you finally understand its worth.
And in a world obsessed with panic, perfection, and performance?
That kind of calm is rare.
That kind of presence is powerful.
That's your edge.

Power That Doesn't Advertise.

Your power isn't always obvious.
You don't need a genius IQ.
You don't need a perfect plan.
You don't need a trust fund, a mentor, or a moment of divine clarity.
You just need to stop dismissing what you've been through.
Because those things that nearly wrecked you?
They were sharpening you.

Every sleepless night.
Every overdraft.
Every funeral.
Every rejection.
Every time you had to smile when your insides were hollow.
Those weren't wasted moments.
They were shaping muscle.
Mental.
Emotional.
Spiritual.
Layer by layer, without applause, without validation, without witnesses.
You were becoming battle-tested in silence.
While others were performing, you were transforming.
While they were chasing aesthetics, you were building endurance.
You're not behind.
You're not cursed.
You're not unlucky.
You've just been training differently.
You've just been building superpowers the hard way.
The kind forged under weight.
The kind that doesn't fade when the spotlight moves on.
And the best part?
No one can take them from you.
They're not rented.
They're not gifted.
They're earned.
Grief gave you perspective.
Struggle gave you hunger.
Rivalry gave you drive.
Put those three together?
That's a fucking weapon.
So no, you're not broken.
You're built.
And if the world doesn't get that yet?
Let them catch up.
You've already lapped them once in silence, now it's time to start showing them why.
Not with noise.

Not with proof.
But with action so undeniable, they'll wish they'd paid attention sooner.

Put It On the Table.

Does this 'thought' hit home?
☐ Yes   ☐ Not really

If yes, can you call yourself out and apply it?
☐ Yes   ☐ Still hiding

If yes, what's one move you'll make to prove it's not just words?

....

....

Thought 44
Feedback Is a Gift.

Most people say they want to get better.
Fitter, sharper, stronger, more successful.
But the moment someone gives them honest feedback?
They shrink.
The air changes.
The walls go up.
Suddenly, the person who *"wanted to improve"* wants to argue instead.
If you can't take feedback, you're not serious about growth.
You're serious about comfort.

Feedback is a fucking mirror.
And most people are terrified of mirrors that show more than their jawline.

We've Confused Support with Softness.

We live in a world where people think being kind means being nice.
That support means sugar-coating.
That growth can be cuddled into existence.
Comfortable.
But wrong.
Support means giving a shit about someone's potential more than their feelings.
It's loving them enough to risk them being pissed at you.
It's valuing their future over their temporary comfort.
And sometimes, that means saying things that sting.

Not to wound them, but to wake them the fuck up.
Because what's worse-hurting their ego for five minutes, or letting them rot in mediocrity?
I'll take a savage truth from someone who wants me to win over a polite lie from someone who just wants me to like them.
Every time.

I Still Remember the One That Stung.

I was pitching for a project.
I thought I'd absolutely nailed it.
My slides were on point.
My lines were polished.
I even threw a shirt on.
I came off the call buzzing.
Then my business partner called me for a debrief.
"Look," he said, *"if I didn't know you, I'd think you were full of shit."*
Silence.
That kind of silence where you can hear your heartbeat in your teeth.
He didn't mean it with malice.
He meant it with love.
And he was right.
I was performing, not connecting.
Chatting in digital jargon, peacocking, and not being real.
What my business partner said shifted everything.
I went back to the drawing board, tore the pitch apart, rewrote it like I was talking to one person I actually gave a damn about.
Landed the client.
Still have them.
That's the power of feedback.
When it's sharp, when it's clean, when it cuts deep enough to draw something better out of you.

Taking Feedback Is a Skill.

It's not natural.

It's not comfortable.
Your instincts will fight it.
Your ego will throw a tantrum.
But it's trainable.
Like a muscle you've never used-awkward at first, then part of your strength.
Next time someone gives you feedback, shut your mouth.
Open your ears.
Breathe through the sting.
Ask yourself - *"What's true here, even if it hurts?"*
Don't defend.
Don't deflect.
Extract.
Find the gold, even if it's covered in shit.
Because the truth is, you can't see your own blind spots.
You're too close to your own noise.
And someone else's perspective might be the thing that unlocks your next level.

The Voice Inside Isn't Always Your Coach.

Not all feedback comes from outside.
Sometimes the loudest critic is living rent-free in your own head.
That voice that says you're not ready.
Not good enough.
Not like them.
It wears the voice of your past.
A parent.
A teacher.
A moment you froze and never forgot.
The rule is - if it's cruel without being useful, it's not a coach.
It's a saboteur.
Real feedback, even when it's internal, has direction.
It shows you the weakness and the way through it.
It doesn't just yell *"you fucking suck"* and walk away.
The rest?
Just noise.

Learn to listen.
Learn to filter.
And if the voice in your head wouldn't dare speak to someone you love that way, tell it to fuck the fuck off.
Twice, if you have to.

Giving Feedback Is a Weapon.

Some people spray opinions like a dog marking territory.
Marking everything in sight, convinced that volume equals value.
Others stay silent when they should speak, letting people drive straight into a wall because *"it's not their place."*
Neither are useful.
Neither help the mission.
Giving feedback is an art.
A skill.
A fucking responsibility.
You're not there to tear someone down.
You're not there to soften the blow until it becomes meaningless.
You're there to be honest, useful, and direct.
Sharp enough to cut through ego but precise enough not to kill the drive.
A real one gives feedback with care - because you want them to win.
With clarity - no fluff, no riddles.
With courage - even if it makes things awkward.
And if they twitch?
Let them.
If they hate you for a minute?
So be it.
Because if they're real, they'll come back stronger.

The Difference Between Critics and Coaches.

There's a big difference between people who want to help you and people who want to hurt you.
Critics shout from the cheap seats.

They don't know you.
They haven't done what you're trying to do.
They couldn't survive one round in your fight.
They don't matter.
Their noise is just that - noise.
Coaches get in the ring.
They've seen your fight.
They believe in your potential.
And they give you the kind of feedback that hurts now but heals later.
Learn to tell the difference.
And when you find a real coach?
Don't run from them.
Sit at their feet and take notes.

You Can't Grow Without Friction.

Muscles grow from tension.
Steel is forged in heat.
And people?
People grow from being challenged.
That's why feedback is a gift - even if it comes wrapped in discomfort.
It shows you care.
It shows someone else cares.
It shows there's more in the tank, and now you know where to look.
You're not being attacked.
You're being invited to level up.
The question is, do you want to?

Real Ones Tell the Truth.

Let me tell you what I value most in the people I keep close -

Radical candour.

The ability to say the uncomfortable thing with love behind it.

The courage to speak truth into someone else's blind spot and not stutter.
If you've got people in your life who do that, hold onto them.
If you don't?
Be that person for someone else.
And if you can't take feedback without melting - grow the fuck up.
Because the people who win long-term?
They seek feedback.
They invite challenge.
They unwrap every uncomfortable truth like it's a golden ticket.
Because they know that next uncomfortable truth might be the one that changes everything.

The Dick-Out Dilemma

Let's keep it simple for the slow learners at the back.
You're walking down the street.
Your zipper's wide open.
Your cock's hanging out.
One of three things is going to happen.

1. People point and laugh, take a picture, maybe post it online.
2. People walk past silently, shake their heads, laugh behind your back.
3. A real one taps you on the shoulder and says - *"The mouse is out of the house."*

Which one do you want?
Exactly.
Be the shoulder tapper.
Thank the shoulder tapper.
And never be the guy walking around with his dick out wondering why life feels cold.

Put It On the Table.

Does this 'thought' hit home?
□ Yes □ Not really

If yes, can you call yourself out and apply it?
□ Yes □ Still hiding

If yes, what's one move you'll make to prove it's not just words?

....

....

Thought 45
Cheap Praise Builds Fragile People.

We live in an era soaked in participation trophies.
Show up?
Congrats, here's your dopamine hit.
Didn't win?
Fuck it, here's a ribbon for trying.
Posted a selfie?
There's your hundred likes and a comment from your mum telling you how *"handsome and successful"* you look.
This isn't encouragement.
It's sedation.
This constant drip-feed of praise is breeding people who believe applause should come standard.
That effort deserves celebration regardless of outcome.
That trying is enough.
It's not.
Acknowledgment isn't the same as achievement.
Validation isn't value.
And a follower count isn't proof of mastery.
If you need praise to proceed, you're not built to survive the storm.

You're Not a Hero for Doing What You're Supposed to Do.

You woke up before sunrise?
Good.
You hit the gym?

Great.
You stuck with your craft for another day?
Solid.
But guess what?
That's not heroic.
That's the bare fucking minimum.
That's table stakes baby.
The price of entry.
You wouldn't congratulate a fish for swimming, so don't expect a standing ovation for doing what you're supposed to do.
Doing your job doesn't make you exceptional.
It makes you functional.
You want to be something rare?
Do it without needing a round of applause.
Do it when no one sees you.
Do it when no one posts about it.
Because legends aren't born in spotlights, they're carved in shadows.

The Silent Killer of Growth.

Clap addiction.
The thirst for applause.
The hunger for likes.
The craving for recognition just for showing up.
If your output depends on being seen, you're not building - you're performing.
That's not work.
That's theatre.
Real growth happens away from the crowd.
In the late hours.
In the grind when your name isn't trending.
In the pain no one praises.
In the quiet that feels like exile but is really incubation.
Clap addiction poisons your drive.
You begin to equate visibility with value.
The real ones don't feed on claps.
They feast on quiet progress.

They stack wins in the dark and don't flinch when the room's empty.
Because they're not chasing noise.
They're chasing improvement.

Praise Is Like Sugar.

Sure, a little encouragement goes a long way.
We all need sparks.
A nod from someone you respect can feel like rocket fuel.
But if you're living off compliments, you're starving your resilience.
If praise is your fuel, what happens when the pump runs dry?
You'll hesitate.
You'll stall.
You'll rot in the silence.
You'll start blaming others for not noticing you.
You'll start expecting rewards for the mere act of existing.

The world doesn't operate on kindness.
It runs on outcomes.
Rewarding results, not intentions.
Nobody owes you applause.
Nobody cares how hard it felt.
What matters is what you built.

Earn Your Own Damn Applause.

You want approval?
Get it from the mirror.
You know what's heavier than public praise?
The private knowledge that you didn't fold.
That you didn't give up.
That you walked through hell with your hands steady.
That's the stuff real pride is made of.
Claps fade.
The crowd moves on to the next shiny thing.
But self-respect?

That's the one audience that never leaves.
It's not about being seen - it's about knowing you didn't take the shortcut.
You didn't make excuses.
You didn't water it down.
And that's worth more than a stadium full of cheers.

Stop Rewarding Mediocrity.

We're stuck in this loop where no one wants to challenge anyone.
No one wants to call bullshit when they see it.
"You tried, that's enough."
"You're doing your best."
"It's okay not to push too hard."
Stop chatting breeze.
Not everyone is doing their best.
Some people are coasting.
Some are hiding behind soft language and softer standards.
Mediocrity thrives when it's coddled.
You want to level up?
Get around people who expect more.
People who don't sugar-coat.
Who don't hand out praise like it's free samples.
People who look at your wins and say -
"Nice, now go harder."
That's love.
That's respect.
That's real.
Because cheap praise isn't a gift, it's a leash.
It teaches you to settle.
To expect more for less.
To stop stretching.

Break that pattern.
Set the bar so high you have to grow just to touch it.
You want to be unshakable?
Then stop craving celebration for surviving.

Survival is the baseline bro.
Build when no one's watching.
Push when no one's clapping.
And let your results make the fucking noise.

Comfort is a Cage.

Comfort kills more dreams than failure ever could.
Praise makes it worse, it gives you a false sense of progress.
You think you're climbing when really, you're just spinning in place.
Clapping hands echo, but they don't push you forward.
Growth feels like pain.
It feels like isolation.
It feels like sacrifice without recognition.
If it feels easy, you're probably not levelling up - you're looping.
Playing the same safe game in a slightly different room.
Get addicted to the burn, not the applause.
Get high on the hard reps.
Get obsessed with the days that leave you drained but proud - the
kind of exhaustion that whispers - *"We're getting somewhere."*
Because when it's all said and done, no one will remember how many
likes you got.
They won't remember your viral post or your perfectly curated bullshit.
They'll remember what you stood for.
What you built.
What you refused to compromise on.
So shut the noise.
Cancel the parade.
Reject the gold stars and the soft pats.
You're not here to be celebrated.
You're here to become something dangerous.
Earn your edge.
In the silence.
In the work.
And when the clapping finally comes, if it comes, let it be an
afterthought not the aim.

Put It On the Table.

Does this 'thought' hit home?
☐ Yes   ☐ Not really

If yes, can you call yourself out and apply it?
☐ Yes   ☐ Still hiding

If yes, what's one move you'll make to prove it's not just words?

....

....

Part 5

LEGACY MODE

Thought 46
Stop Chasing Trends - Be the Standard.

Every time you chase what's popular, you hand over your power. You start trimming your edges to fit the current shape.
You trade clarity for clout.
You put on a mask and hope no one sees the hesitation underneath.
You wear shoes that don't fit just because they're trending.
You shape your voice to echo the latest buzz, hoping to be accepted.
And what happens?
You disappear.
You fade into the feed.
You become one more filter on a recycled loop.
You start competing for scraps of attention from people who never gave a shit about you in the first place.
You become the thing you once promised you'd never be - a watered-down version of someone else.
A second-hand echo.
A ghost in your own skin.

"Fuck crossing over to them, let them cross over to us." - N.W.A.

"Me Too" Is a Weak Strategy.

Let's get real.
If your whole move is "me too," you're not just behind, you're beneath.
You're playing on someone else's field, using their ball, their rules, their scoreboard.

You're reacting.
You're chasing.
You're waiting for someone to go first so you can copy without risk.
You speak in the tone of the day.
You dress for the algorithm.
You live for trends that vanish by morning.
You're not building anything.
You're not carving your name into stone.
You're scribbling in sand, wondering why nothing lasts.
People can smell it.
They can feel when there's no soul behind the style.
No core behind the copy.
Because there's no depth in mimicry.
No gravity in imitation.
No thunder in following.

Be So Solid They Have to Adjust to You.

Real ones don't bend to the noise.
They don't edit their voice to fit in.
They don't trim their truth to stay liked.
They double down.
They cement their presence.
"This is how I move.
You want in?
Cross over to me."
That's authority.
That's what N.W.A. understood.
They weren't going to dilute the message for radio play or suburban approval.
They weren't begging for mass appeal.
They knew their sound.
Their mission.
Their purpose.
And because they didn't cross over, others had to.

You want to matter?
Don't shapeshift to survive.
Stand so firmly in who you are that the room has to make space.

Originals Don't Look for Permission.

You don't need anyone's blessing to be who you are.
You need nerve.
You need direction.
You need the guts to keep going when people call you *"too much,"*
"too raw," or *"too intense."*
Originals make the safe crowd squirm.
They break the rhythm people are used to marching to.
They confuse the ones addicted to clones - because realness doesn't
come with a manual.
They draw criticism first.
Then curiosity.
Then followers.
That's the pattern.
Confusion.
Controversy.
Conversion.
But it doesn't happen if you're busy asking for permission.
The moment you wait to be validated, you're already off course.

Why Blend In When You're Built to Stand Out?

Most people blend in not because they believe in the trend but
because they fear the silence that comes with being different.
They're scared of being judged.
Scared of missing the hype.
Scared of standing alone.
The brutal truth?
Waves crash.
Standards last.

Trends spin out.
Moods shift.
But principles?
Those stack.
That's legacy.
Staying true might cost you clout now.
But in the long game, nothing compounds like authenticity.

Set the Vibe, Don't Mirror It.

Let them chase each other in circles.
Let them dilute, repackage, and relabel the same tired ideas.
You?
You build.
You build what's real.
You build what lasts.
You build your own gravity.
When you become the constant in a spinning world, people come to you for stability.
They come to you to recalibrate.
To remember what matters.
To feel something that isn't disposable.
"Fuck crossing over to them, let them cross over to us."
That's not arrogance.
That's position.
That's what happens when your foundation is so firm, others shift their orbit to be near it.

You're Not a Billboard, You're a Beacon.

Trends make you a product.
Standards make you a presence.
Trends treat you like a billboard - visible, replaceable, forgettable.
But when you set the standard, you become a beacon.
You light the path for others to follow.
That takes more than style.

It takes substance.
It takes conviction when it's easier to conform.
So stop tweaking your identity to be digestible.
Stop diluting your message to be shareable, like it's some cheap piece of content.
You're not here to be palatable.
You're here to be unforgettable.

They'll Doubt You Then Copy You.

At first, they'll mock you.
They'll question you.
They'll call you stubborn, arrogant, difficult - all the names people throw when they don't understand what they're looking at.
But when your results start to stack, when your name carries weight, they'll borrow your words.
They'll mimic your moves.
They'll try to steal the blueprint, trace your lines, wear your skin.
Let them.
Because by then, you'll already be onto the next layer.
Already growing beyond their reach.
Already setting the next standard they'll chase.

Trends Are Comfortable. Standards Are Confrontational.

Chasing what's hot is easy.
It keeps you liked.
It keeps you safe.
Setting a standard?
That's a different animal.
That gets you called out.
That gets you misunderstood.
That puts pressure on your every move.
Good.

Pressure reveals truth.
Friction sharpens vision.
If your standard doesn't scare you a little, it's not high enough.
Being the standard means carrying weight - and carrying it well, even when your arms are shaking.
It's the grind that builds muscle nobody can fake.

Don't Cross Over. Call Them Up.

Don't trim your edges just to sit at someone else's table.
Flip the table.
If the room can't handle your truth, it's the wrong room.
If the crowd wants you quiet, speak louder.
If the trend is pulling you sideways, plant your feet.
Be the reason the world adjusts.
Be the voice they didn't know they needed until they heard it.
Be the shape they couldn't categorise but couldn't ignore.
That's power.
That's presence.
That's leadership.

The Cost of Being Unapologetic.

Remember - there's a price for not flinching.
For refusing to shrink.
For showing up without soft edges and without the pre-approved hashtags.
Without the safe little filter that makes you easier to swallow.
And yeah, you'll pay for it.
Not in theory - in real-time.
People won't clap, they'll critique.
They won't lean in, they'll recoil.
They'll question your motives, your tone, your right to stand that tall.
You'll get side-eyed in rooms where you once got applause.
You'll lose followers the second you stop saying what's easy to digest.

You'll be labelled difficult, intense, aggressive, because you didn't put a smiley face on your truth.
That cost is the toll for real impact.
Being unapologetic means owning the whole of who you are, without trying to soften it for approval.
It means walking into rooms and not folding just to make others comfortable.
It means speaking even when your voice shakes, even when you know they'll twist your words before they understand them.
And most people aren't ready for that heat.
So they retreat.
They conform.
They soften to stay 'marketable'.
But not you.
You choose the edge.
You choose clarity over likability.
You choose integrity over trendiness.

That choice will cost you popularity.
You choose the kind of truth that might burn a bridge - but it'll also light the path for the people meant to find you.
That choice will cost you popularity.
It might cost you partnerships.
It might even cost you friendships built on mutual pretending.
But you weren't born to be palatable, you were born to be potent.

They might not get it now.
They might not respect it today.
But one thing's certain - they'll remember it.
Because unapologetic presence lingers.
It echoes in their head long after they've unfollowed you.
It leaves a mark that polished mimicry never could.
So let them label you.
Let them misunderstand.
Let them throw your name around in rooms you've outgrown.
Just don't let them reshape you.
This isn't about arrogance - it's about alignment.
It's about not negotiating your identity for likes.

It's about standing so firm in who you are that the friction becomes fuel.
That's the cost of being unapologetic.
And it's worth every scar.

Anchor Down.

Stop chasing what's next.
Be what lasts.
Stop folding into the crowd.
Be the figure they can't look away from.
Stop crossing over to them.
Build your world brick by brick.
Hold your ground like you've got roots in concrete.
Speak your truth like you've got nothing left to lose.
And let them come to you when they're ready to move different.

Put It On the Table.

Does this 'thought' hit home?
☐ Yes   ☐ Not really

If yes, can you call yourself out and apply it?
☐ Yes   ☐ Still hiding

If yes, what's one move you'll make to prove it's not just words?

....

....

Thought 47
Built for the Back Door.

I was shite at school.
Shite at uni.
Shite at most things, if we're being honest.
Not because I didn't try.
Not because I didn't care.
Because the system was never built for people like me.
I didn't fit.
Didn't think the way they wanted.
Didn't move in neat lines.
Didn't do what I was told unless I saw a reason.
While the so-called smart kids were racking up grades, I was racking up doubts.
Every test I tanked wasn't just a score - it was another voice whispering, *"You're thick.*
You're slow.
You're not one of them."
But I've lived long enough now to see it different.
Turns out, there's more than one way into the building.
Some people walk through the front door in polished shoes with neat little qualifications tucked under their arm.
Me?
I came in through the fire exit, boots muddy, clothes torn, dragging my past like a steel chain.
And I didn't knock.
I kicked it in.

The System Doesn't Want Wild

Schools.
Universities.
Corporate ladders.
They're not built for thinkers.
They're built for box-tickers.
If you're obedient, compliant, and good at repeating back what you're told?
You'll glide through.
But if you question too much...
If you ask "*why*" when silence is expected...
If you twitch at sitting still and ache to move your hands, build things, break things, rewire what's broken...
Then brace yourself.
The system will call you names.
Disruptive.
Lazy.
Hard work.
They won't say - "*You're gifted in a different way.*"
They'll say - "*You're difficult.*"
And that label sticks.
It follows you like a shadow, whispering that you're the problem.
You'll shrink.
Doubt yourself.
Start cutting off parts of who you are just to squeeze into something that never fit.
But the truth?
You're not broken.
You're built for open skies, not small rooms.

I remember struggling with all of this as a kid.
Feeling like I was wired wrong.
Like everyone else got the manual and I missed the memo.
And my dad - in the middle of one of my meltdowns - looked at me and said - "*Son, tame rabbits don't come from wild ones.*"
That stuck.
Because maybe I wasn't supposed to be calm.

Or neat.
Or manageable.
Maybe I was meant to run.

Work That Doesn't Feel Like Work.

Everything shifted the day I stumbled across something that didn't feel like a job.
Not something I was merely good at.
Not something that paid the bills.
Something that made me feel more me.
For me, it was building - businesses, ideas, momentum.
Taking raw sparks from other people's minds and fanning them into flames.
Creating from scratch.
Laying the first brick with shaky hands and still doing it anyway.
Suddenly, I wasn't dragging my feet anymore.
I was sprinting, eyes wild, mind electric.
I didn't need to be told to work harder - I had to be told to stop.
Because when you're in the right lane, the gas pedal's welded to the floor.
And that same brain that failed in school?
It became a weapon.
A heat-seeking missile, locked onto what mattered.
Because when you finally aim your energy at the right target?
You don't just get better.
You become dangerous.

The Lie You've Been Sold.

Most people?
They're asleep.
Sleepwalking through jobs they don't love.
Chasing goals they didn't set.
Living lives that look fine from the outside but feel like sandpaper on the inside.

They're not dead, but they're not alive either..
Ask them why they're doing it and they'll say - *"It's stable."*
"It pays well."
"It's what I've always done."
Bollocks.
That's what happens when you confuse comfort with happiness.
They're not living.
They're surviving.
They've traded purpose for predictability, and they don't even see the bars of the cage anymore.
And you?
You don't need more stuff.
You need something that sets your chest on fire.
You need to be lit the fuck up.

This Is About Survival.

Finding what moves you isn't a cute dream.
It's life or death.
Look around - how many people are bitter?
Tired?
Picking fights over nothing?
It's not random.
It's what happens when you unplug someone from meaning.
They've lost their fire.
And without that spark, even the strongest person will start to fade.
You weren't born to tread water.
You weren't meant to climb someone else's ladder.
You were made to build your own - even if you've got to weld the fucking rungs together with your teeth.
And no, you don't have to be brilliant at it straight away.
You just have to care enough to try.
Because caring is the fuel that keeps you going when nothing else makes sense.
If it matters, you'll learn.
If it fuels you, you'll fail forward until the thing starts to take shape.

One day you'll look up, and without even noticing it, you'll be a decade deep.
And the version of you that once felt small will be long gone.

You Were Never the Problem.

If you've ever been told you were too intense, too sensitive, too slow, too loud, too stubborn...
If you've ever felt like your mind was tuned to a frequency no one else could hear...
Good.
It means you're still connected to something real.
Something the beige, boardroom-approved masses can't touch.
The world isn't built for originals.
It's built for easy-to-sell, easy-to-control replicas.
It rewards obedience, not vision.
It loves predictability more than brilliance.
But replicas don't change anything.
If you don't fit the mould, don't shrink to fit it.
Smash it.
Make your own.

The Back Door Was Always the Way.

You never needed to charm your way through the front.
You never needed approval.
You needed persistence.
You needed to keep knocking until something cracked open.
Or better yet?
Build your own damn door.
And when you finally get through, don't forget who you are.
Don't soften just to blend in.
Stay gritty.
Stay weird.
Stay stubborn.

Because the back door wasn't a shortcut.
It was a trial by fire.
And you survived it.
Now build your table.
Invite the other misfits.
Show them that *"no"* is just another way of saying *"find another way in."*
And remember you were never broken.
You were never behind.
You were just built for the back door.

Put It On the Table.

Does this 'thought' hit home?
☐ Yes   ☐ Not really

If yes, can you call yourself out and apply it?
☐ Yes   ☐ Still hiding

If yes, what's one move you'll make to prove it's not just words?

....

....

Thought 48
The World Doesn't Owe You a Purpose.

Y ou are not special.
You're not owed clarity.
And you are definitely not above the graft.
The world doesn't owe you a dream, a calling, or a clean run at life.
It doesn't owe you a curated existence that 'feels aligned' every fucking day.
But too many people wander through life like the universe is their personal assistant, waiting to be handed a custom-built destiny, tied up with purpose, passion, and their star sign.
Wake up.
That's not how this works.
Life isn't a delivery service.
No one's dropping off meaning at your doorstep.
You get what you grind for.
And if you're sat waiting for fate to hand you the keys?
You'll be waiting forever.

Purpose Isn't Found. It's Built.

You don't stumble across purpose like it's spare change down the back of the sofa.
You forge it.
You pick something.
You give a shit.
You commit.

Then you show up when it's tedious.
When it's thankless.
When no one's clapping.
You keep showing up.
And one day, that thing you stuck with?
It starts to shape you.
Not because it was handed to you but because you carved it from sweat and bloody-mindedness.

Entitlement Is a Disease.

Know what really winds me up?
People who reckon they're too good to start small.
Too talented to fail.
Too brainy to get their hands dirty.
Too visionary to finish what they started.
That's not hunger.
That's ego.
And ego will starve you.
You're not better than the process.
You're not exempt from effort.
You're not above the grind - you're just scared of being humbled by it.
Nobody cares how much potential you've got if it's all talk.
That's the poison of entitlement - it convinces you that dreaming big is enough.
It's not.
You want to lead?
Show up and take the hits.
You want respect?
Deliver something that costs you.
You want meaning?
Bleed for it.
No shortcuts.
No one's coming to validate your ambition.
You earn it, or you don't get it.

No Purpose Without Responsibility.

You'll never touch meaning if you keep dodging responsibility.
Responsibility is weighty.
It's messy, draining, uncomfortable.
But it's the threshold.
The moment you take charge of something - your health, your work,
your people, your story - you begin to anchor identity.
And from identity, you forge purpose.
It doesn't come from chasing freedom - it comes from showing up
even when freedom sounds easier.
Purpose lives where commitment begins.
And commitment starts the moment you stop looking for the exit.

You Don't Need to Be Inspired, You Need to Move.

The inspiration junkies are everywhere.
Living off podcasts, reels, and self-help fluff that makes them feel
good but does nothing.
They're waiting for the perfect quote.
The lightning bolt.
That magic phrase that'll unlock them.
Newsflash -
You're not 'the one' until you do the bloody work.
You don't need another reel.
You need to move.
Start.
Get it wrong.
Fix it.
Keep going.
Meaning isn't in your mood board.
It's in your movement.

You're Not Better Than Anyone.

Think you're above others?

You've already lost.
Arrogance is a slow leak in your potential.
But humility?
That's fuel.
Wake up and ask - *"How can I sharpen today?"*
"Where can I take proper ownership?"
"What's one thing I'll finish with care, no shortcuts?"
That's dangerous thinking.
Because most people are too busy curating an image.
Pretending to have it all figured out.
You?
You're building something real.
Quiet.
Relentless.
Unshakeable.

Build It.
Bleed for It.
Own It.
There's no map coming.
No golden envelope marked - 'Your Purpose.'
What you get is today.
So choose.
Commit.
Fuck it up.
Own it.
Come back stronger.
And keep swinging.
Until one day, you'll look around and realise - this thing you've built?
It's not just what you do.
It's who you are.
That's purpose.
And it's yours.
Because no one gave it to you.
And no one can take it away.
The world doesn't owe you purpose.
But you owe it to yourself to build one that matters.

Put It On the Table.

Does this 'thought' hit home?
☐ Yes   ☐ Not really

If yes, can you call yourself out and apply it?
☐ Yes   ☐ Still hiding

If yes, what's one move you'll make to prove it's not just words?

....

....

Thought 49
Legacy Isn't a Statue, It's the Ripples You Leave.

A sudden goodbye.
On 2nd September 2021, I learned what legacy really means. My dad, known to many as Hoppy, drove himself to A&E, thinking he just had a stubborn stomach cramp.
Typical of him - strong, private, independent - didn't want to make a fuss.
By the evening, everything changed.
The doctors pulled us aside.
Terminal liver cancer.
Maybe 24 hours left.
No one prepares you for a countdown that short.
The air gets heavy.
He was transferred to The Christie.
My mother, my brothers, and I stayed by his bedside for three days, listening to James Taylor, Coldplay, and Cara Dillon.
There was no grand ending.
No last monologue.
Just silence.
One moment he was here.
The next, a hole opened in the world.
My best friend and mentor.
Gone.

But in that hollow space, something stirred.
It wasn't just grief.
It was presence.
Energy.

As if he'd left behind something that couldn't die.
I could feel it in conversations with people he'd helped.
In the way others moved, worked, gave, because of him.
His story hadn't ended.
It was still unfolding.
Through people.
Through action.
Through echoes.
That's when I realised, legacy isn't about what stands still.
It's about what keeps moving.

The Man Called Hoppy.

He wasn't famous.
You won't find his name on plaques or statues.
But if you looked closer - in youth clubs, in broken systems he patched up, in tired kids who found hope - you'll find him everywhere.
He was a fundraiser.
A fixer.
A mentor who didn't care for pleasantries but gave a damn in all the ways that mattered.
When the system failed someone, he became the system.
If there was a gap, he filled it with his own two hands.
He saw need, and instead of asking why someone else hadn't stepped in, he stepped up.
Again.
And again.
No drama.
No spotlight.
Just relentless generosity, stitched together with grit.
He told the truth, even when it stung.
Especially when it stung.
But if he called you out, he also had your back.
He could challenge you and still be your biggest ally in the same breath.

His life's work?

Helping kids.
Not with empty promises, but with real resources, hard-won funding, and opportunities they'd never have got otherwise.
One night, he helped raise over a million pounds.
The next morning, he was already planning the next project.
He didn't coast on yesterday's wins.
He moved.
"*Acta non verba*" he used to say.
Actions not words.

He didn't chase fame.
His reward was in kids who had futures they wouldn't otherwise have.
Fellow fundraisers called him a hero, a coach, a mentor.
For some, he was the reason they stepped into charity work.
For others, especially the overlooked and the struggling - he was the reason they still had hope.
No one will see his name in lights.
But his fingerprints are all over lives.

No Statue, Only Ripples.

Legacy is what people do because you lived.
I feel dad when I walk into youth clubs he helped build.
In the kids who didn't fall through the cracks because he caught them.
In the mentors who now give because he once gave to them.
He never got to see all his seeds bloom - one youth centre he'd poured himself into opened only after he passed.
He never saw the doors swing open.
But his DNA was on every wall.
I've walked the corridors of Warrington Youth Zone and felt like he was two steps ahead of me, pointing things out.
That's the thing about ripples.
You don't always see how far they travel.
But they move.
And they keep moving.

The Real Measure.

Legacy isn't defined by long eulogies.
It lives in quiet habits.
In words that echo.
In values that refuse to die.
I hear him in my own voice when I'm mentoring someone.
When I speak the same truth he once spoke to me - firm but full of care.
I see him in the way I choose to show up, especially when it's inconvenient.

He built more than projects.
He built people.
That's the stuff that lasts.

Make Ripples That Last.

We like to tell ourselves legacy is for the extraordinary.
The geniuses.
The saints.
The billionaires.
Bullshit.
Legacy's for anyone who decides to care consistently.
You don't need to save the world.
You need to show up for it.
Start small.
A kind word.
A moment of patience.
A refusal to turn away when it's easier to stay uninvolved.
One gesture.
One shift.
One drop in the still water.
Here's how you begin - focus on people, not praise.
The loudest echoes often come from the quietest actions.
Be consistent.

Anyone can show up once, but legacy is built by those who show up daily.
Pass on your values.
Be someone your younger self needed.
Be someone your future self can be proud of.
Think beyond your timeline.
Plant trees you'll never sit beneath.
Invest in futures you might never witness.
You don't need to be perfect.
You need to be present.
Because every act you make out of love or grit or justice leaves a mark. Whether or not you see it, that mark stays.
It moves.
It carries.

A Ripple Can Save a Life.

One word of encouragement.
One moment of belief in someone who's lost it.
One opportunity given when it wasn't deserved but was desperately needed.
That can change a direction.
Break a cycle.
Save a life.
That's not hyperbole - that's how this works.
We think legacy has to be grand, visible, undeniable.
But sometimes the most powerful ripples are the ones you'll never trace back to yourself.
So ask yourself, what ripples will I leave?
You don't need a roadmap.
You don't need a master plan.
You need to take the next right step - with honesty, with fire, and with heart.
That daily choice?
It will echo further than you think.
When you hold the door open.
When you lift someone up.

When you call someone in.
When you refuse to let a good person give up on themselves.
That ripple moves.
And long after you're gone, those moments might still be shaping lives.
That's what Hoppy showed me.
Not with a speech.
Not with a script.
But with how he lived - and how he left.
He set off waves.
And now, I get to keep them moving.
So do you.
You don't need permission.
You don't need perfection.
You just need heart.
The only legacy that matters is the one that ripples on without you.
Start now.

The Weight of Carrying It Forward.

When someone like Hoppy goes, the world expects a baton to be passed.
And I feel that - not as pressure, but as responsibility.
Not to mimic him, but to honour what he stood for.
I know where my strengths lie.
And where they don't.
I'm not going to raise a million quid in 24 hours - that was his game.
Mine looks different.
And that's exactly the point.
My legacy, and honouring his, isn't about repeating tactics.
It's about continuing principles.
Kindness and grit.
That's the spine I try to carry into everything I do.
I think about it constantly - in how I treat people, how I show up, how I lead, how I speak.
Even writing this book is part of it.

Someone once asked me - "*Why are you writing a book?*"
My answer was simple - "*I want to change a life.*"
That's it.
One life.
One underdog.
One person who connects with one of these 'thoughts' and decides to commit to change.
That's how I create a ripple.

Hoppy and Me by Zak.

"*I remember it as if it was yesterday. A thirteen-year-old, struggling and scared, was asked to speak about my life and my love for movies at an annual charity gala chaired by Nichols PLC. Nervous, tense, I remember walking through Mere Country Club to do my rehearsal. I waited with bated breath in the lobby until a man, adorned in a bodacious shirt/kilt combo approached me, with the warmest of smiles and an even warmer embrace.*
That was Hoppy. The man who sat with me after knowing me for all of 5 minutes, and treated me as if I was an old friend. I vividly recall him telling me, "Fuck the crowds. It's all noise. But you're the king, and they're here for you."

Thereon, Hoppy would continue to gleefully, proudly follow me in between the shadows. Always checking up on me through connections at Warrington Youth Club (now Youth Zone).

Things came to a heartbreaking halt when, a day after my 21st birthday, I was told he wasn't well. And days later, Hoppy left this world. With all the love, peace, and power in his heart. With the biggest impact on millions of people, businesses and charities - but with the greatest impact any human being had ever had on little old me.

I made the choice that every decision I make from that day, is a "What would Hoppy do?"

And if we do a Christopher Nolan for a moment and flash forward, I find myself as a filmmaker, writing and directing real movies, with my own crew, with a bachelor's degree in Filmmaking, with a beautiful girlfriend, and find myself working in the Youth Zone that he fought tooth and nail to set up and a dream that he kept alive and still keeps alive long after his passing. I work in that building, and I teach young people how to make films! Because I want to help those kids who were once like me, in those similar predicaments, I want to be the beam of light for those kids that Hoppy was (and still very, very much is), for me.

I miss him always. A tear daily is shed when I routinely listen to Jerusalem and Sky Full of Stars, and he may not be there to see these things and to impact those things in my life anymore.

And he may have missed my directorial debut, but damn it - he didn't.

He lives in everything I do.

You magnificent genius. I miss you." - Zak Cameron

Put It On the Table.

Does this 'thought' hit home?
☐ Yes   ☐ Not really

If yes, can you call yourself out and apply it?
☐ Yes   ☐ Still hiding

If yes, what's one move you'll make to prove it's not just words?

....

....

Thought 50
The Wild Pig Doesn't Wait for Permission.

Here it is.
The end of the road.
Except it's not.
Not really.
Because if you've made it this far, you already know this book was never meant to be read and filed away.
It was meant to start something.
To light the fuse.
You've just been handed the match.
What you do with it now?
That's on you.

No One Is Coming to Save You.

There is no grand unveiling.
No knighting ceremony.
No perfect moment when someone taps you on the shoulder and says -
"You're ready now."
No mentor.
No partner.
No parent.
No guru.
No green light.
You're already holding the keys.
You just need to stop asking for permission to use them.

Stop waiting.
Stop stalling.
Stop polishing your potential like it's something that needs to be perfect before it's real.
Waiting is a lie dressed up as preparation.
Stillness is fear in a suit.
You are not a child hoping to be picked for the team - you are the team.
You are the shot-caller.
You are the fucking wild pig.
And wild pigs?
They don't wait.
They charge.

Permission Is the Cage. Action Is the Key.

You want to write a book?
Write the first page.
Want to change your body?
Lace up.
Want to start a business?
Sell something.
Anything.
Today.
Action is your way out.
It's ugly.
It's messy.
It's loud.
But it works.
You already know what to do.
If you're brutally honest, you've known for a while.
You just haven't trusted yourself to start.
So trust.
Not in perfection.
In movement.
Belief doesn't come first.
Action does.

And action builds belief the way bricks build a home - one hard, heavy, deliberate piece at a time.

They're Not Watching You Like You Think.

Your brain lies to you.
Tells you the world is watching, judging, waiting for you to fuck up.
The truth is that everyone else is too busy drowning in their own doubt to give a shit about what you're doing.
They're not watching you.
They're watching themselves.
So fall.
Fuck up.
Miss the mark.
And then get back up faster than you went down.
Because the only thing more unforgettable than failure is resilience.

Be the Fire, Not the Fan.

This world is full of spectators.
Clappers.
Critics.
Commentators.
People with opinions but no skin in the game.
People who measure their worth by how loudly they can point out your flaws.
They'll boo at your start.
They'll mock your momentum.
They'll cheer if you stop.
Let them.
Because you weren't built for the stands.
You weren't built to blend.
Light your own fire.
Let it rage.
Let it burn every fucking bridge that leads back to the old you.

This Book Ends. But You Don't.

This is the final page.
But not the final word.
You don't need another line, another quote, another plan.
You need to move.
You need to run headfirst into the thing that scares you most.
Because you're not made for the waiting room.
You're made for the wild.
So here it is - your permission slip.
Go.
And don't stop until the ground shakes.

www.ingramcontent.com/pod-product-compliance
Ingram Content Group UK Ltd.
Pitfield, Milton Keynes, MK11 3LW, UK
UKHW040746131025
8354UKWH00028B/112